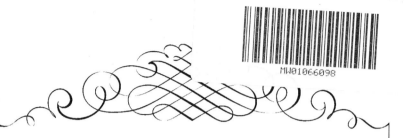
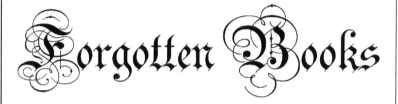
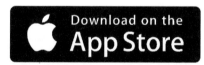
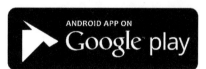

ISBN 978-1-331-18101-9
PIBN 10154960

1 MONTH OF
FREE
READING

at

www.ForgottenBooks.com

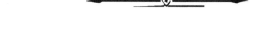

By purchasing this book you are eligible for one month membership to ForgottenBooks.com, giving you unlimited access to our entire collection of over 700,000 titles via our web site and mobile apps.

To claim your free month visit:

www.forgottenbooks.com/free154960

SLEEP

AND

ITS DERANGEMENTS.

BY

WILLIAM A. HAMMOND, M.D.,

PROFESSOR OF DISEASES OF THE MIND AND NERVOUS SYSTEM, AND OF CLINICAL MEDICINE
IN THE BELLEVUE HOSPITAL MEDICAL COLLEGE, NEW YORK; VICE-PRESIDENT OF
THE ACADEMY OF THE MEDICAL SCIENCES, NATIONAL INSTITUTE
OF LETTERS, ARTS, AND SCIENCES; LATE SURGEON-
GENERAL U. S. ARMY, ETC. ETC.

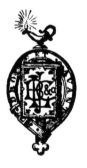

PHILADELPHIA:

J. B. LIPPINCOTT & CO.

1869.

PREFACE.

THE basis of this little volume is a paper on Insomnia, published in the New York Medical Journal in May and June, 1865. This was subsequently enlarged and published in a separate form, under the title "Wakefulness, with an Introductory Chapter on the Physiology of Sleep."

The very favorable reception which it met with in this country, in Great Britain, and on the Continent, from the medical press, the profession, and the public generally, led to the exhaustion of a large edition in a few months.

The present issue was announced nearly two years ago, and the printing begun. Increasing professional duties have, however, prevented me bestowing that continuous labor upon it which was desirable, and hence the publication has been long delayed. My

1*   (v)

J82

apologies therefore are due, first, to my excellent
and dear friend, the senior member of the house of
J. B. Lippincott & Co., whose patience I know
has been severely tried, but who has scarcely reproached me for my neglect; and second, to that
portion of the public which has been kind enough
to make repeated inquiries relative to the appearance of this monograph, and which I trust will not
be disappointed, now that it is really published.

162 WEST 34TH ST., NEW YORK,
July 10*th*, 1869.

CONTENTS.

(vii)

CHAPTER IX.

CHAPTER X.

CHAPTER XI.

CHAPTER XII.

SLEEP AND ITS DERANGEMENTS.

CHAPTER I.

THE NECESSITY FOR SLEEP.

THE state of general repose which accompanies sleep is of especial value to the organism in allowing the nutrition of the nervous tissue to go on at a greater rate than its destructive metamorphosis. The same effect is, of course, produced upon the other structures of the body; but this is not of so much importance as regards them, for while we are awake they all obtain a not inconsiderable amount of rest. Even those actions which are most continuous, such as respiration and the pulsation of the heart, have distinct periods of suspension. Thus, after the contraction and dilatation of the auricles and ventricles of the heart, there is an interval during which the organ is at rest. This amounts to one-fourth of the time requisite to make one pulsation and begin another. During six hours of the twenty-four the heart is, therefore, in a state of complete equal parts, one will be occupied in inspiration, one in expiration, and the other by a period of quiescence. During eight hours of the day, therefore, the muscles of respiration and the lungs are inactive. And so with the several glands. Each has its time for rest. And of the voluntary muscles, none, even during our most untiring waking moments, are kept in continued action.

But for the brain there is no rest, except during sleep, and even this condition is, as we all know, only one of comparative quietude in many instances. So long as an individual is awake, there is not a single second of his life during which the brain is altogether inactive; and even while he is deprived by sleep of the power of volition, nearly every other faculty of the mind is capable of being exercised; and several of them, as the imagination and memory, for instance, are sometimes carried to a pitch of exaltation not ordinarily reached by direct and voluntary efforts. If it were not for the fact that all parts of the brain are not in action at the same time, and that thus some slight measure of repose is afforded, it would probably be impossible for the organ to maintain itself in a state of integrity.

During wakefulness therefore the brain is constantly in action, though this action may be of such a character as not always to make us conscious of its performance. A great deal of the power of the brain is expended in the continuance of functional operations necessary to our well-being. During sleep these

are altogether arrested or else very materially retarded in force and frequency.

Many instances of what Dr. Carpenter very happily calls "unconscious cerebration" will suggest
themselves to the reader. We frequently find suggestions occurring to us suddenly—suggestions
which could only have arisen as the result of a train
of ideas passing through our minds, but of which
we have been unconscious. This function of the
brain continues in sleep, but not with so much force
as during wakefulness. The movements of the heart,
of the inspiratory muscles, and of other organs which
perform either dynamic or secretory functions are
all rendered less active by sleep; and during this
condition the nervous system generally obtains the
repose which its ceaseless activity during our periods
of wakefulness so imperatively demands. Sleep is
thus necessary in order that the body, and especially
the brain and nervous system, may be renovated by
the formation of new tissue to take the place of that
which by use has lost its normal characteristics.

From what has been said it will be seen that the
brain is no exception to the law which prevails
throughout the whole domain of organic nature—
that use causes decay. The following extract from
another work* bears upon this point, and I think
tends to its elucidation.

"During life the fluids and tissues of the body are

---

* See the author's Treatise on Hygiene, page 92.

constantly undergoing change. New matter is deposited, and the old is removed with ceaseless activity. The body may be regarded as a complex machine, in which the law, that force is only generated by decomposition, is fully carried out. Every motion of the body, every pulsation of the heart, every thought which emanates from the encephalon is accompanied by the destruction of a certain amount of tissue. As long as food is supplied in abundance, and the assimilative functions are not disordered, reparation proceeds as rapidly as decay, and life is the result; but should nutrition be arrested, by any cause, for any considerable period, new matter ceases to be formed, and the organs, worn out, act no longer, and death ensues.

"The animal body differs from any inorganic machine in the fact that it possesses the power of self-repair. In the steam-engine, for instance, the fuel which serves for the production of steam, and subsequently for the creation of force, can do nothing toward the repair of the parts which have been worn out by use. Day by day, by constant attrition and other causes, the engine becomes less perfect, and eventually must be put in order by the workman. In the animal body, however, the material which serves for the production of force is the body itself, and the substances which are taken as food are assimilated according to their character by those organs and parts which require them.

"The body is therefore undergoing continued

change. The hair of yesterday is not the hair of to-day; the muscle which extends the arm is not identically the same muscle after as before its action; old material has been removed and new has been deposited to an equal extent; and though the weight and form, the chemical constitution and histological character have been preserved, the identity has been lost."

All this is especially true of the brain. Its substance is consumed by every thought, by every action of the will, by every sound that is heard, by every object that is seen, by every substance that is touched, by every odor that is smelled, by every painful or pleasurable sensation, and so each instant of our lives witnesses the decay of some portion of its mass and the formation of new material to take its place. The necessity for sleep is due to the fact that during our waking moments the formation of the new substance does not go on as rapidly as the decay of the old. The state of comparative repose which attends upon this condition allows the balance to be restored, and hence the feeling of freshness and rejuvenation we experience after a sound and healthy sleep. The more active the mind the greater the necessity for sleep, just as with a steamer, the greater the number of revolutions its engine makes, the more imperative is the demand for fuel.

The power with which this necessity can act is oftentimes very great, and not even the strongest exertion of the will is able to neutralize it. I have frequently seen soldiers sleep on horseback during night marches, and have often slept thus myself. Galen on one occasion walked over two hundred yards while in a sound sleep. He would probably have gone farther but for the fact of his striking his foot against a stone and thus awaking.

The Abbé Richard states that' once when coming from the country alone and on foot, sleep overtook him when he was more than half a league from town. He continued to walk, however, though soundly asleep, over an uneven and crooked road.*

Even when the most stirring events are transpiring, some of the participants may fall asleep. Sentinels on posts of great danger cannot always resist the influence. To punish a man with death, therefore, for yielding to an inexorable law of his being, is not the least of the barbarous customs which are still in force in civilized armies. During the battle of the Nile many of the boys engaged in handing ammunition fell asleep, notwithstanding the noise and confusion of the action and the fear of punishment. And it is said that on the retreat to Corunna whole battalions of infantry slept while in rapid march. Even the most acute bodily sufferings are not always sufficient to prevent sleep. I have seen individuals who had been exposed to great fatigue, and who had while enduring it met with accidents requiring surgical interference, sleep

* La Théorie des Songes. Paris, 1766, p. 206.

through the pain caused by the knife. Damiens, who attempted the assassination of Louis XV. of France, and who was sentenced to be torn to pieces by four horses, was for an hour and a half before his execution subjected to the most infamous tortures, with red-hot pincers, melted lead, burning sulphur, boiling oil, and other diabolical contrivances, yet he slept on the rack, and it was only by continually changing the mode of torture, so as to give a new sensation, that he was kept awake. He complained, just before his death, that the deprivation of sleep was the greatest of all his torments.

Dr. Forbes Winslow* quotes from the *Louisville Semi-Monthly Medical News* the following case:

"A Chinese merchant had been convicted of murdering his wife, and was sentenced to die by being deprived of sleep. This painful mode of death was carried into effect under the following circumstances: The condemned was placed in prison under the care of three of the police guard, who relieved each other every alternate hour, and who prevented the prisoner falling asleep night or day. He thus lived nineteen days without enjoying any sleep. At the commencement of the eighth day his sufferings were so intense that he implored the authorities to grant him the blessed opportunity of being strangled, guillotined, burned to death, drowned, garroted,

---

* On Obscure Diseases of the Brain, etc. London, 1860, p. 604, note.

shot, quartered, blown up with gunpowder, or put to death in any conceivable way their humanity or ferocity could invent. This will give a slight idea of the horrors of death from want of sleep."

In infants the necessity for sleep is much greater than in adults, and still more so than in old persons. In the former the formative processes are much more active than those concerned in disintegration. Hence the greater necessity for frequent periods of repose. In old persons, on the contrary, decay predominates over construction, there is a decreased activity of the brain, the nervous system, and of all other organs, and thus the demand for rest and recuperation is lessened.

The necessity for sleep is not felt by all organic beings alike. The differences observed are more due to variations in habits, modes of life, and inherent organic dispositions, than to any inequality in the size of the brain, although the latter has been thought by some authors to be the cause. It has been assumed that the larger the brain the more sleep was required. Perhaps this is true as regards the individuals of any one species of animals, but it is not the case when species are compared with each other. In man, for instance, persons with large heads, as a rule, have large, well-developed brains, and consequently more cerebral action than individuals with small brains. There is accordingly a greater waste of cerebral substance and an increased necessity for repair.

This is not, however, always the case, as some individuals with small brains have been remarkable for great mental activity.

All animals sleep, and even plants have their periods of comparative repose. As Lelut says :*

"No one is ignorant of the nocturnal repose of plants. I say repose and nothing else. I do not say diminution or suspension of their sensibility, for plants have no sensibility. I say diminution of their organic actions—a diminution which is evident and characteristic in all, more evident and more characteristic in some. * * *

"Their interior or vital movements are lessened, the flow of the sap and of other fluids which penetrate and rise in them is retarded. Their more mobile parts—the leaves, the flowers—show by their falling, their occlusion, their inclination that their organic actions are diminished, and that a kind of repose has been initiated, which takes the place of the lying down, which, with animals, is the condition and the result of sleep."

---

* Physiologie de la Pensée. Recherche Critique des Rapports du Corps à l'Esprit. Deuxième édition. Paris, 1862, t. ii. p. 440.

CHAPTER II.

THE CAUSES OF SLEEP.

THE exciting cause of natural and periodic sleep is undoubtedly to be found in the fact that the brain at stated times requires repose, in order that the cerebral substance which has been decomposed by mental and nervous action may be replaced by new material. There are other exciting causes than this, however, for sleep is not always induced by ordinary or natural influences acting periodically. There are many others, which within the strict limits of health may cause such a condition of the brain as to produce sleep.

Authors, in considering sleep, have not always drawn the proper distinction between the exciting and the immediate cause. Thus Macario,* in alluding to the alleged causes of sleep, says:

"Among physiologists some attribute it to a congestion of blood in the brain; others to a directly opposite cause, that is, to a diminished afflux of blood to this organ; some ascribe it to a loss of nervous

---

* Du Sommeil, des Rêves et du Somnambulisme, etc. Lyon, 1857, p. 14.

fluid, others to a flow of this fluid back to its source; others again find the cause in the cessation of the motion of the cerebral fibers, or rather in a partial motion in these fibers. Here I stop, for I could not, even if I wished, mention all the theories which have prevailed relative to this subject. I will only add that, in my opinion, the most probable proximate and immediate cause appears to be feebleness. What seems to prove this view is the fact that exhaustive hot baths, heat, fatigue, too great mental application are among the means which produce sleep."

Undoubtedly the influence mentioned by Macario, and many others which he might have cited, lead to sleep. They do so through the medium of the nervous system—causing a certain change to take place in the physical condition of the brain. We constantly see instances of this transmission of impressions and the production of palpable effects. Under the influence of fatigue, the countenance becomes pale; through the actions of certain emotions, blushing takes place. When we are anxious or suffering or engaged in intense thought, the perspiration comes out in big drops on our brows; danger makes some men tremble, grief causes tears to flow. Many other examples will suggest themselves to the reader. It is surely, therefore, no assumption to say that certain mental or physical influences are capable of inducing such an alteration in the state of the brain as necessarily to cause sleep. These influences or exciting causes I propose to consider in detail, after having given my views relative to the condition of the brain which immediately produces sleep.

It is well established as regards other viscera, that during a condition of activity there is more blood in their tissues than while they are at rest. It is strange, therefore, that, relative to the brain, the contrary doctrine should have prevailed so long, and that even now, after the subject has been so well elucidated by exact observation, it should be the generally received opinion that during sleep the cerebral tissues are in a state approaching congestion. Thus Dr. Marshall Hall,* while contending for this view, also advances the theory that there is a special set of muscles, the duty of which is, by assuming a condition of tonic contraction, so to compress certain veins as to prevent the return of the blood from the heart.

Dr. Carpenter† is of the opinion that the first cause of sleep in order of importance is the pressure exerted by distended blood-vessels upon the encephalon.

Sir Henry Holland‡ declares that a " degree of pressure is essential to perfect and uniform sleep."

Dr. Dickson§ regards an increased determination

---

* Observations in Medicine.   Second Series, p. 27.

† Art. *Sleep*. Cyclopedia of Anatomy and Physiology, vol. iv. part 1, p. 681.

‡ Chapters on Mental Physiology.   London, 1852, p. 105.

§ Essays on Life, Sleep, Pain, etc.   Philadelphia, 1852, pp. 63 and 64.

of blood to the cerebral mass, and its consequent congestion in the larger vessels of the brain, as necessary to the induction of sleep.

In his very excellent work on Epilepsy, Dr. Sieveking* says:

"Whether or not there is actually an increase in the amount of blood in the brain during sleep, and whether, as has been suggested, the choroid plexuses become turgid or not, we are unable to affirm otherwise than hypothetically; the evidence is more in favor of cerebral congestion than of the opposite condition inducing sleep—evidence supplied by physiology and pathology." Dr. Sieveking does not, however, state what this evidence is.

Barthez† is of the opinion that during sleep there is a general plethora of the smaller blood-vessels of the whole body. He does not appear to have any definite views relative to the condition of the cerebral circulation.

Cabanis‡ declares that as soon as the necessity for sleep is experienced, there is an increased flow of blood to the brain.

To come to more popular books than those from which we have quoted, we find Mr. Lewes,§ when

---

* Epilepsy and Epileptiform Seizures. London, 1858, p. 123.

† Nouveaux Éléments de la Science de l'Homme 3me édition. Paris, 1858, vol. ii p. 7, et seq

‡ Rapports du Physique et du Morale de l'Homme. Paris, 1824, p. 379.

§ The Physiology of Common Life. New York, 1860, vol. ii. p. 305.

speaking of the causes of sleep, asserting that: "It is caused by fatigue, because one of the natural consequences of continued action is a slight congestion; and it is the *congestion* which produces sleep. Of this there are many proofs." Mr. Lewes omits to specify these proofs.

Macnish* holds the view that sleep is due to a determination of blood to the head.

That a similar opinion has prevailed from very ancient times, it would be easy to show. I do not, however, propose to bring forward any further citations on this point, except the following, from a curious old black-letter book now before me, in which the views expressed, though obscure, are perhaps as intelligible as many met with in books of our own day:

"And the holy scripture in sundrie places doth call death by the name of sleepe, which is meant in respect of the resurrection; for, as after sleepe we hope to wake, so after death we hope to rise againe. But that definition which Paulus Ægineta maketh of sleepe, in my judgment, is most perfect where he saith: Sleepe is the rest of the pores animall, proceeding of some profitable humour moistening the braine. For here is shewed by what means sleepe is caused; that is, by vapours and fumes rising from the stomache to the head, where through coldness of the braine they being congealed, doe stop the

---

* Philosophy of Sleep.   Second edition, 1850, p. 5.

conduites and waies of the senses, and so procure
sleepe, which thing may plainly be perceived here-
by; for that immediately after meate we are most
prone to sleepe, because then the vapours ascende
most abundantly to the braine, and such things as
be most vaporous do most dispose to sleepe, as wine,
milke, and such like."*

The theory that sleep is due directly to pressure
of blood-vessels, filled to repletion, upon the cerebral tissues, doubtless originated in the fact that a
comatose condition may be thus induced. This
fact has long been known. Servetus, among other
physiological truths, distinctly announces it in his
Christianismi Restitutio, when he says:

" *Et quando ventriculi ita opplentur pituita, ut arteriæ
ipsæ choroidis ea immergantur, tunc subito generatur ap-
poplexia.*"

Perhaps the theory which prevails at present, of
sleep being due to the pressure of distended blood-
vessels upon the choroid plexus, is derived from
these words of Servetus.

That stupor may be produced by pressure upon
the brain admits of no doubt. It is familiarly
known to physicians, surgeons, and physiologists;
the two former meet with instances due to pathological causes every day, and the latter bring it on

* The Haven of Health, chiefly made for the comfort of Students,
and consequently for all those that have a care for their health, etc.
By Thomas Cogan, Master of Arts and Batchelor of Physic. London,
1612, p. 332.

at will in their laboratories. But this form of coma and sleep are by no means identical. On the contrary, the only point of resemblance between the two consists in the fact that both are accompanied by a loss of volition. It is true, we may often arrive at a correct idea of a physiological process from determining the causes and phenomena of its pathological variations, but such a course is always liable to lead to great errors, and should be conducted with every possible precaution. In the matter under consideration it is especially of doubtful propriety, for the reason stated, that coma is not to be regarded as a modification of sleep, but as a distinct morbid condition. Sir T. C. Morgan,* in alluding to the fact that sleep has been ascribed to a congested state of the brain, for the reason that in apoplectic stupor the blood-vessels of that organ are abnormally distended, objects to the theory, on the ground that it assimilates a dangerous malady to a natural and beneficial process. He states (what was true at the time he wrote) that the condition of the circulation through the brain, during sleep, is wholly unknown.

It is important to understand clearly the difference between stupor and sleep, and it is very certain that the distinction is not always made by physicians; yet the causes of the two conditions have

---

* Sketches of the Philosophy of Life. London, 1819, p 262.

almost nothing in common, and the phenomena of each are even more distinct.

1. In the first place, stupor never occurs in the healthy individual, while sleep is a necessity of life.

2. It is easy to awaken a person from sleep, while it is often impossible to arouse him from stupor.

3. In sleep the mind may be active, in stupor it is as it were dead.

4. Pressure upon the brain, intense congestion of its vessels, the circulation of poisoned blood through its substance cause stupor, but do not induce sleep. For the production of the latter condition a diminished supply of blood to the brain, as will be fully shown hereafter, is necessary.

Perhaps no one agent so distinctly points out the difference between sleep and stupor as opium and its several preparations. A small dose of this medicine acting as a stimulant increases the activity of the cerebral circulation, and excites a corresponding increase in the rapidity and brilliancy of our thoughts. A larger dose lessens the amount of blood in the brain, and induces sleep. A very large dose sometimes diminishes the power of the whole nervous system, lessens the activity of the respiratory function, and hence allows blood which has not been properly subjected to the influence of the oxygen of the atmosphere to circulate through the vessels of the brain. There is nothing in the opium itself which produces excitement, sleep, or stupor, by any direct action upon the brain. All its effects are due

3

to its influence on the heart and blood-vessels
through the medium, however, of the nervous system.   This point can be made plainer by adducing
the results of some experiments which I have lately
performed.

Experiment.—I placed three dogs of about the same
size under the influence of chloroform, and removed
from each a portion of the upper surface of the skull
an inch square.   The dura mater was also removed,
and the brain exposed.   After the effects of the
chloroform had passed off—some three hours subsequent to the operation—I administered to number
one the fourth of a grain of opium, to number two
a grain, and to number three two grains.   The brain
of each was at the time in a perfectly natural condition.

At first the circulation of the blood in the brain
was rendered more active, and the respiration became more hurried.   The blood-vessels, as seen
through the openings in the skulls, were fuller and
redder than before the opium was given, and the
brain of each animal rose through the hole in the
cranium.   Very soon, however, the uniformity which
prevailed in these respects was destroyed.   In number one the vessels remained moderately distended
and florid for almost an hour, and then the brain
slowly regained its ordinary appearance.   In number
two the active congestion passed off in less than half
an hour, and was succeeded by a condition of very
decided shrinking, the surface of the brain having

fallen below the surface of the skull, and become pale. As these changes supervened, the animal gradually sank into a sound sleep, from which it could easily be awakened. In number three the surface of the brain became dark, almost black, from the circulation of blood containing a super-abundance of carbon, and owing to diminished action of the heart and vessels it sank below the level of the opening, showing, therefore, a diminished amount of blood in its tissue. At the same time the number of respirations per minute fell from 26 to 14, and they were much weaker than before. A condition of complete stupor was also induced from which the animal could not be aroused. It persisted for two hours. During its continuance, sensation of all kind was abolished, and the power of motion was altogether lost.

It might be supposed that the conditions present in numbers two and three differed only in degree. That this was not the case is shown by the following experiment:

Experiment.—To the dogs two and three I administered on the following day, as before, one and two grains of opium respectively. As soon as the effects began to be manifested upon the condition of the brain, I opened the trachea of each, and, inserting the nozzle of a bellows, began the process of artificial respiration. In both dogs the congestion of the blood-vessels of the brain disappeared. The brain became collapsed, and the animals fell into a sound

sleep, from which they were easily awakened. If
the action of the bellows was stopped and the animals were left to their own respiratory efforts, no
change ensued in number two, but in number three
the surface of the brain became dark, and stupor
resulted.

In order to be perfectly assured upon the subject,
I proceeded as follows with another dog:

Experiment.—The animal was trephined as was the
others, and five grains of opium given. At the same
time the trachea was opened and the process of artificial respiration instituted. The brain became
slightly congested, then collapsed, and sleep ensued.
The sleep was sound, but the animal was easily
awakened by tickling its ear. After I had continued
the process for an hour and a quarter, I removed the
nozzle of the bellows, and allowed the animal to
breathe for itself. Immediately the vessels of the
brain were filled with black blood, and the surface
of the brain assumed a very dark appearance.

The dog could no longer be aroused, and died one
hour and a quarter after the process was stopped.

I have only stated those points of the experiments
cited which bear upon the subject under consideration, reserving for another occasion others of great
interest. It is, however, shown that a small dose of
opium excites the mind, because it increases the
amount of blood in the brain; that a moderate dose
causes sleep, because it lessens the amount of blood;
and that a large dose produces stupor by impeding

the respiratory process, and hence allowing blood loaded with carbon, and therefore poisonous, to circulate through the brain.

It is also shown that the condition of the brain during stupor is very different from that which exists during sleep. In the one case its vessels are loaded with dark blood; in the other they are comparatively empty, and the blood remains florid.

I think it will be sufficiently established, in the course of these remarks, that sleep is directly caused by the circulation of a less quantity of blood through the cerebral tissues than traverses them while we are awake. This is the immediate cause of healthy sleep. Its exciting cause is, as we have seen, the necessity for repair. The condition of the brain which is favorable to sleep may also be induced by various other causes, such as heat, cold, narcotics, anæsthetics, intoxicating liquors, loss of blood, etc. If these agents are allowed to act excessively, or others, such as carbonic oxide, and all those which interfere with the oxygenation of the blood, are permitted to exert their influence, stupor results.

The theory above enunciated, although proposed in a modified form by Blumenbach several years since, and subsequently supported by facts brought forward by other observers, has not been received with favor by any considerable number of physiologists. Before, therefore, detailing my own experience, I propose to adduce a few of the most striking proofs of its correctness which I have been able to collect, together with the opinions of some of those inquirers who have recently studied the subject from this point of view.

Blumenbach* details the case of a young man, eighteen years of age, who had fallen from an eminence and fractured the frontal bone, on the right side of the coronal suture. After recovery took place a hiatus remained, covered only by the integument. While the young man was awake this chasm was quite superficial, but as soon as sleep ensued it became very deep. The change was due to the fact that during sleep the brain was in a collapsed condition. From a careful observation of this case, as well as from a consideration of the phenomena attendant on the hibernation of animals, Blumenbach† arrives at the conclusion that the proximate cause of sleep consists in a diminished flow of oxygenated blood to the brain.

Playfair‡ thinks that sleep is due to "a diminished supply of oxygen to the brain."

Dendy§ states that there was, in 1821, at Montpellier, a woman who had lost part of her skull, and the brain and its membranes lay bare. When she was in deep sleep the brain remained motionless beneath the crest of the cranial bones; when she was

---

* Elements of Physiology. Translated by John Elliotson, M D., etc. 4th edition. London, 1828, p. 191.

† Op. cit. p. 282, et seq.

‡ Northern Journal of Medicine, No. 1, 1844, p. 34.

§ The Philosophy of Mystery. London, 1841, p. 283.

dreaming it became somewhat elevated; and when she was awake it was protruded through the fissure in the skull.

Among the most striking proofs of the correctness of the view that sleep is due to diminished flow of blood to the head, are the experiments of Dr. Alexander Fleming,* late Professor of Medicine, Queen's College, Cork. This observer states, that while preparing a lecture on the mode of operation of narcotic medicines, he conceived the idea of trying the effect of compressing the carotid arteries on the functions of the brain. The first experiment was performed on himself, by a friend, with the effect of causing immediate and deep sleep. The attempt was frequently made, both on himself and others, and always with success "A soft humming in the ears is heard; a sense of tingling steals over the body, and in a few seconds complete unconsciousness and insensibility supervene, and continue so long as the pressure is maintained."

Dr. Fleming adds, that whatever practical value may be attached to his observations, they are at least important as physiological facts, and as throwing light on the causes of sleep. It is remarkable that his experiments have received so little notice from physiologists.

Dr. Bedford Brown,† of North Carolina, has re-

---

* British and Foreign Medico-Chirurgical Review, Am. ed., April, 1855, p. 404.

† American Journal of the Medical Sciences, October, 1860, p. 399.

corded an interesting case of extensive compound fracture of the cranium, in which the opportunity was afforded him of examining the condition of the cerebral circulation while the patient was under the influence of an anæsthetic, preparatory to the operation of trephining being performed. A mixture of ether and chloroform was used. Dr. Brown says:

"Whenever the anæsthetic influence began to subside, the surface of the brain presented a florid and injected appearance. The hemorrhage increased, and the force of the pulsation became much greater. At these times so great was the alternate heaving and bulging of the brain, that we were compelled to suspend operations until they were quieted by a repetition of the remedy. Then the pulsations would diminish, the cerebral surface recede within the opening of the skull, as if by collapse; the appearance of the organ becoming pale and shrunken with a cessation of the bleeding. In fact, we were convinced that diminished vascularity of the brain was an invariable result of the impression of chloroform or ether. The changes above alluded to recurred sufficiently often, during the progress of the operation, in connection with the anæsthetic treatment, to satisfy us that there could be no mistake as to the cause and effect."

It will be shown, in the course of the present memoir, that Dr. Brown's conclusions, though in the main correct, are erroneous so far as they relate to the effect of chloroform upon the cerebral circulation; nor does it appear that he employed this agent unmixed with ether, in the case which he has recorded so well. He has, probably, based his remarks on this point upon the phenomena observed when the compound of ether and chloroform was used— the action of pure chloroform, as regards its effect upon the quantity of blood circulating through the brain, being the reverse of that which he claims for it.

But the most philosophical and most carefully digested memoir upon the proximate cause of sleep, which has yet been published, is that of Mr. Durham.* Although my own experiments in the same direction, and which will be hereafter detailed, were of prior date, I cheerfully yield all the honor which may attach to the determination of the question under consideration to this gentleman, who has not only worked it out independently, but has anticipated me several years in the publication, besides carrying his researches to a much further point than my own extended.

With the view of ascertaining by ocular examination the vascular condition of the brain during sleep, Durham placed a dog under the influence of chloroform, and removed with a trephine a portion of bone as large as a shilling from the parietal region; the dura mater was also cut away. During

---

* The Physiology of Sleep. By Arthur E. Durham. Guy's Hospital Reports, 3d Series, vol. vi. 1860, p. 149.

the continuance of the anæsthetic influence, the large veins of the surface of the pia mater were distended, and the smaller vessels were full of dark-colored blood. The longer the administration of the chloroform was continued, the greater was the congestion. As the effects of this agent passed off, the animal sank into a natural sleep, and then the condition of the brain was very materially changed. Its surface became pale and sank down below the level of the bone; the veins ceased to be distended, and many which had been full of dark blood could no longer be distinguished. When the animal was roused, the surface of the brain became suffused with a red blush, and it ascended into the opening through the skull. As the mental excitement increased, the brain became more and more turgid with blood, and innumerable vessels sprang into sight. The circulation was also increased in rapidity. After being fed, the animal fell asleep, and the brain again became contracted and pale. In all these observations the contrast between the two conditions was exceedingly well marked.

To obviate any possible effects due to atmospheric pressure, watch-glasses were applied to the opening in the skull, and securely cemented to the edges with Canada balsam. The phenomena observed did not differ from those previously noticed; and, in fact, many repetitions of the experiment gave like results.

Durham, in the next place, applied ligatures to the jugular and vertebral veins, with the effect—as was to be expected—of producing intense congestion of the brain, attended with coma. This last condition he very properly separates from sleep, which is never caused by pressure from the veins. He likens sleep to the state induced by preventing the access of blood to the brain through the carotids, but does not allude to Fleming's researches on this point.

From his observations, Durham deduces the following conclusions:

" 1. Pressure of distended veins upon the brain is not the cause of sleep, for during sleep the veins are not distended; and when they are, symptoms and appearances arise which differ from those which characterize sleep.

" 2. During sleep the brain is in a comparatively bloodless condition, and the blood in the encephalic vessels is not only diminished in quantity, but moves with diminished rapidity.

" 3. The condition of the cerebral circulation during sleep is, from physical causes, that which is most favorable to the nutrition of the brain tissue; and, on the other hand, the condition which prevails during waking is associated with mental activity, because it is that which is most favorable to oxydation of the brain substance, and to various changes in its chemical constitution.

" 4. The blood which is derived from the brain during sleep is distributed to the alimentary and excretory organs.

" 5. Whatever increases the activity of the cerebral circulation tends to preserve wakefulness; and whatever decreases the activity of the cerebral circulation, and, at the same time, is nòt inconsistent with the general health of the body, tends to induce and favor sleep. Such circumstances may act primarily through the nervous or through the vascular system. Among those which act through the nervous system, may be instanced the presence or absence of impressions upon the senses, and the presence or absence of exciting ideas. Among those which act through the vascular system, may be mentioned unnaturally or naturally increased or decreased force or frequency of the heart's action.

"6. A probable explanation of the reason why quiescence of the brain normally follows its activity, is suggested by the recognized analogical fact that the products of chemical action interfere with the continuance of the action by which they are produced."

Luys,* after stating the two opposite views relative to the state of the cerebral circulation during sleep, gives his adhesion on principles of analogy to that which holds to a diminished afflux of blood. Taking the condition of the salivary glands during their periods of inaction as the basis of his argument, he says:

"We are then naturally led, in making the application of known facts to those which are yet un-

---

* Recherches sur la Système Nerveux Cerebro-Spinal, sa Structure, ses Fonctions et ses Maladies. Paris, 1865, p. 448.

known, to say that the nervous tissue and the gland-ular tissue present, between themselves, the closest analogy, so far as circulatory phenomena and the double alternation of their periods of activity and repose are concerned. And that if the period dur-ing which the gland reconstitutes its immediate principles corresponds to a period of reduced activ-ity of circulatory phenomena—to a state of relative anæmia—and that when it functionates it is awak-ened to a state in which its capillaries are turgid with blood, it is very admissible that the same circulatory conditions should be present in the nervous tissue, and that the period of inactivity, or of sleep, should be characterized by an anemic state. Inversely, the period of activity or wakefulness should be marked by an acceleration of the flow of blood, and by a kind of erethism of the vascular element."

Having thus, in as succinct a manner as possible, brought forward the principal observations relative to the immediate cause of sleep, which up to the present time have been published, I come, in the next place, to detail the result of my own researches.

In 1854 a man came under my observation who had, through a frightful railroad accident, lost about eighteen square inches of his skull. There was thus a fissure of his cranium three inches wide and six inches long. The lost portion consisted of a great part of the left parietal, and part of the frontal, oc-cipital, and right parietal bones. The man, who was employed as a wood chopper, was subject to severe

4*

and frequent epileptic fits, during which I often attended him. In the course of my treatment, I soon became acquainted with the fact that, at the beginning of the comatose condition which succeeded the fits, there was invariably an elevation of that portion of the scalp covering the deficiency in the cranium. As the stupor passed away, and sleep from which he could easily be aroused ensued, the scalp gradually became depressed. When the man was awake, the region of scalp in question was always nearly on a level with the upper surface of the cranial bones. I also noticed on several occasions that during natural sleep the fissure was deeper, and that in the instant of awaking, the scalp covering it rose to a much higher level.

After my attention was thus drawn to this subject, I observed that in young infants the portion of scalp covering the anterior fontanelle was always depressed during sleep, and elevated during wakefulness.

During the summer of 1860 I undertook a series of experiments, with the view of ascertaining the condition of the cerebral circulation during sleep, of which the following is a brief abstract:

A medium-sized dog was trephined over the left parietal bone, close to the sagittal suture, having previously been placed under the full anæsthetic influence of ether. The opening made bv the trephine was enlarged with a pair of strong bone-forceps, so as to expose the dura mater to the extent of a full square inch. This membrane was then cut away

and the brain brought into view. It was sunk below
the inner surface of the skull, and but few vessels
were visible. Those which could be perceived, however, evidently conveyed dark blood, and the whole
exposed surface of the brain was of a purple color.
As the anæsthetic influence passed off, the circulation of the blood in the brain became more active.
The purple hue faded away, and numerous small
vessels filled with red blood became visible; at the
same time the volume of the brain increased, and
when the animal became fully aroused, the organ
protruded through the opening in the skull to such
an extent that, at the most prominent part, its surface was more than a quarter of an inch above the
external surface of the cranium. While the dog
continued awake, the condition and position of the
brain remained unchanged. After the lapse of half
an hour, sleep ensued. While this state was coming
on I watched the brain very attentively. Its volume
slowly decreased; many of its smaller blood-vessels
became invisible, and finally it was so much contracted that its surface, pale and apparently deprived
of blood, was far below the level of the cranial wall.

Two hours subsequently the animal was again
etherized, in order that the influence of the ether
upon the cerebral circulation might be observed
from the commencement. At the time the dog was
awake, and had a few minutes previously eaten a
little meat and drank a small quantity of water. The
brain protruded through the opening in the skull,

and its surface was of a pink hue, with numerous red vessels ramifying over it. The ether was administered by applying to the muzzle of the animal a towel folded into the shape of a funnel, and containing a small sponge saturated with the agent.

As soon as the dog commenced to inspire the ether, the appearance of the brain underwent a change of color, and its volume became less. As the process of etherization was continued, the color of the surface darkened to a deep purple, and it ceased to protrude through the opening. Finally, when a state of complete anæsthesia was reached, it was perceived that the surface of the brain was far below the level of the cranial fissure, and that its vessels conveyed black blood alone.

Gradually the animal regained its consciousness; the vessels resumed their red color, and the brain was again elevated to its former position. In this last experiment there did not appear to be any congestion of the brain. Had this condition existed, it would have been difficult to account for the diminntion in bulk, which certainly took place. There was evidently less blood in the cerebral tissue than there had been previously at the etherization; but this blood, instead of being oxygenated, was loaded with excrementitial matters, and consequently was not fitted to maintain the brain in a condition of activity.

The following morning, the dog being quite lively, I removed the sutures which had been placed in the skin, covering the hole in the cranium, with the view of ascertaining the effects of chloroform upon the brain, when introduced into the system by inhalation. Suppuration had not yet taken place, and the parts were in good condition. The opening in the skull was completely filled by the brain, and the surface of the latter was traversed by a great many small vessels carrying red blood. The chloroform was administered in the same way in which the ether had been given the previous day.

In a few seconds the change in color of the blood circulating in the vessels began to take place, but there was no sinking of the brain below the level of the chasm in the skull. On the contrary, its protrusion was greater than before the commencement of the experiment. There was thus not only unoxygenated blood circulating to too great an extent through the brain, but there was very decided congestion.

The foregoing experiments were frequently repeated on other dogs, and also on rabbits, with like results. Within a short period I have in part gone over the ground again, without observing any essential point of difference in the effects produced.

I have never repeated Fleming's experiment on the human subject, except in one instance, and then sleep, or a condition resembling it, was instantaneously produced. As soon as the pressure was removed from the carotids, the individual gained his consciousness. On dogs and rabbits, however, I have performed it frequently, and though if the pres-

sure be continued for longer than one minute, convulsions generally ensue, a state of insensibility resembling natural sleep is always the first result.
Lately, I have had, through the kindness of my
friend, Dr. Van Buren, the opportunity of examining a case which affords strong confirmation of the
correctness of the preceding views. It was that of a
lady in whom both common carotids were tied for a
cirsoid aneurism, involving a great portion of the
right side of the scalp. One carotid was tied by the
late Dr. J. Kearney Rogers, and the other by Dr.
Van Buren, seven years ago, with the effect of ar-
resting the progress of the disease. No peculiar
symptoms were observed in consequence of these
operations, except the supervention of persistent
drowsiness, which was especially well marked after
the last operation, and which, even now, is at times
quite troublesome.

We thus see that the *immediate* cause of sleep is a
diminution of the quantity of blood circulating in
the vessels of the brain, and that the *exciting* cause
of periodical and natural sleep is the necessity which
exists that the loss of substance which the brain has
undergone, during its state of greatest activity,
should be restored. To use the simile of the steam-
engine again, the fires are lowered and the opera-
tives go to work to repair damages and put the machine in order for next day's work.

Whatever other cause is capable of lessening the
quantity of blood in the brain is also capable of in-

ducing sleep. There is no exception to this law, and hence we are frequently able to produce this condition at will. Several of these factors have been already referred to, but it will be interesting to consider them all somewhat more at length.

Heat.—Most persons in our climate, and in those of higher temperatures, have felt the influence of heat in causing drowsiness, and eventually sleep, if the action is powerful enough and sufficiently prolonged. It is not difficult to understand the mode by which heat acts in giving rise to sleep. During the prevalence of high temperatures the blood flows in increased proportion to the surface of the body and to the extremities, and consequently the quantity in the brain is diminished. Sleep accordingly results unless the irritation induced by the heat is so great as to excite the nervous system. Heat applied directly to the head exerts, of course, a directly contrary effect upon the cerebral circulation, as we see in sun-stroke. Here there is internal cerebral congestion, loss of consciousness, stupor, etc.

That the effect of heat is to dilate the vessels of the part subjected to its influence, can be ascertained by putting the arm or leg into hot water. The swelling of the blood-vessels is then very distinctly seen. It will be shown hereafter that one of the best means of causing sleep in morbid wakefulness is the warm-bath.

Cold.—A slight degree of cold excites wakefulness

at first, but if the constitution be strong the effect is
to predispose to sleep. This it does by reason of
the determination of blood to the surface of the body
which moderate cold induces in vigorous persons.
The ruddy complexion and warmth of the hands
and feet produced in such individuals under the
action of this influence are well known.

But if the cold be very intense, or the reduction
of temperature sudden, the system, even of the
strongest persons, cannot maintain a resistance, and
then a very different series of phenomena result.
Stupor, not sleep, is the consequence. The blood-
vessels of the surface of the body contract and the
blood accumulates in the internal organs, the brain
among them. Many instances are on record showing the effect of extreme cold in producing stupor
and even death. One of the most remarkable of
these is that related by Captain Cook, in regard to
an excursion of Sir Joseph Banks, Dr. Solander,
and nine others, over the hills of Terra del Fuego.
Dr. Solander, knowing from his experience in
Northern Europe that the stupor produced by severe cold would terminate in death unless resisted,
urged his companions to keep in motion when they
began to feel drowsy. "Whoever sits down will
sleep," said he, "and whoever sleeps will rise no
more." Yet he was the first to feel this irresistible
desire for repose, and entreated his companions to
allow him to lie down. He was roused from his
stupor with great difficulty and carried to a fire,

when he revived. Two black men of the party, whose organizations were not so robust as those of the whites, perished. Dr. Whiting* relates the case of Dr. Edward Daniel Clark, the celebrated traveler, who on one occasion came very near losing his life by cold. He had performed divine service at a church near Cambridge, and was returning home on horseback, when he felt himself becoming very cold and sleepy. Knowing the danger of yielding to the influence which was creeping over him, he put his horse into a fast trot, hoping thereby to arouse himself from the alarming torpor. This means proving unavailing, he got down and led his horse, walking as fast as he could. This, however, did not long succeed. The bridle dropped from his arm, his legs became weaker and weaker, and he was just sinking to the ground when a gentleman who knew him came up in a carriage and rescued him.

I have often myself noticed this effect of cold in producing numbness and drowsiness, and on one occasion was nearly overcome by it. I was crossing the mountain ridge between Cebolleta and Covero, in New Mexico, when the thermometer fell in about two hours from 52° to 22° Fahrenheit. So great was the effect upon me that if I had had much farther to go I should probably have succumbed. As it was, I reached a rancho in time to be relieved, though several minutes elapsed before I was able to

---

* Cyclopedia of Practical Medicine, article *Cold*.

speak. The sensations experienced were rather agreeable than otherwise. There was a great desire to rest and to yield to the languor which was present, and there was a feeling of recklessness which rendered me perfectly indifferent to the consequences. I should have dismounted from my horse and given way to the longing for repose if I had been able to do so. I have several times experienced very similar effects from change of air. A few years since I was so drowsy at the sea-coast, whither I had gone from a hot city, that it was with difficulty I could keep awake, even when engaged in active physical exercise.

Another potent cause of sleep, and one of which we generally avail ourselves, is the *diminution of the power of the attention*. To bring this influence into action generally requires only the operation of the will under circumstances favorable to the object in view. Shutting the eyes so as to exclude light, getting beyond the sound of noises, refraining from the employment of the other senses, and avoiding thought of all kind, will generally, when there is no preventing cause, induce sleep. To think, and to maintain ourselves in connection with the outward world by means of our senses requires that the circulation of blood in the brain shall be active. When we isolate ourselves from external things, and restrain our thoughts, we lessen the amount of blood in the brain, and sleep results. It is not, however, always easy for us to do this. The nervous system is excited, ideas follow each other in rapid succession, and we lie awake hour after hour vainly trying to forget that we exist. The more the will is brought to bear upon the subject the more rebellious is the brain, and the more it will not be forced by such means into a state of quietude. We must then either let it run riot till it is worn out by its extravagancies, or we must fatigue it by requiring it to perform labor which is disagreeable. Just as we might do with an individual of highly destructive propensities, who was going about pulling down his neighbors' houses. We might, if we were altogether unable to stop him, let him alone till he had become thoroughly wearied with his exertions, or we might divert him from his plan by guiding him to some tough piece of work which would exhaust his strength sooner than would his original labor.

Many ways of thus tiring the brain have been proposed. The more irksome they are, the more likely they are to prove effectual. Counting a hundred backward many times, listening to monotonous sounds, thinking of some extremely disagreeable and tiresome subject, with many other devices, have been suggested, and have proved more or less effectual. Boerhaave* states that he procured sleep by placing a brass pan in such a position that the patient heard the sound of water which was made to

---

* Cyclopedia of Anatomy and Physiology, vol. iv., part 1, p. 681, article *Sleep*.

fall into it, drop by drop. In general terms, monot-
ony predisposes to sleep. Dr. Dickson* quotes
Southey's experience as related in the Doctor,† and
I also cannot do better than lay it before the reader,
particularly as it indicates several methods which
may be more efficacious with others than the one he
found to succeed so admirably.

"I put my arms out of bed; I turned the pillow
for the sake of applying a cold surface to my cheek;
I stretched my feet into the cold corner; I listened
to the river and to the ticking of my watch; I
thought of all sleepy sounds and of all soporific
things—the flow of water, the humming of bees,
the motion of a boat, the waving of a field of corn,
the nodding of a mandarin's head on the chimney-
piece, a horse in a mill, the opera, Mr. Humdrum's
conversations, Mr. Proser's poems, Mr. Laxative's
speeches, Mr. Lengthy's sermons. I tried the de-
vice of my own childhood, and fancied that the bed
rushed with me round and round. At length Mor-
pheus reminded me of Dr. Torpedo's Divinity Lectures, where the voice, the manner, the matter, even
the very atmosphere and the streamy candlelight
were all alike somnific; when he who, by strong
effort, lifted up his head and forced open the reluctant eyes never failed to see all around him asleep.
Lettuces, cowslip wine, poppy syrup, mandragora,

* Essays on Life, Sleep, and Pain. Philadelphia, 1852, p. 87.
† The Doctor, etc., edited by Rev. John Wood Warter. London.

hop pillows, spider's web pills, and the whole tribe of narcotics, up to bang and the black-drop, would have failed,—but this was irresistible; and thus, twenty years after date, I found benefit from having attended the course."

Frequently the power of the attention is diminished by natural causes. After the mind has been strained a long time in one particular direction, and during which period the brain was doubtless replete with blood, the tension is at last removed, the blood flows out of the brain, the face becomes pale, and sleep ensues. It is thus, as Macnish* says, that "the finished gratification of all ardent desires has the effect of inducing slumber; hence after any keen excitement the mind becomes exhausted and speedily relapses into this state."

A gentleman recently under my care for a paralytic affection, informed me that he could at any time render himself sleepy by looking for a few minutes at a bright light, so as to fatigue the eyes, or by paying particular attention to the noises in the street, so as to weary the sense of hearing. It is well known that sleep may be induced by gentle frictions of various parts of the body, and doubtless the other senses are capable of being so exhausted, if I may use the expression, as to diminish the power of the attention, and thus lessen the demand for blood in the brain. As a consequence, sleep ensues.

* Op. c t , p. 5.

5

The cutting off of sensorial impressions aids in lessening the power of the attention and thus predisposes to sleep. Stillness, darkness, the absence of any decided impression on the skin, and the non-existence of odors and flavors, accomplish this end. In these respects, however, habit exercises great influence, and thus individuals, for instance, who are accustomed to continual loud noises, cannot sleep when the sound is interrupted. As we have already seen, however, the predisposition to sleep is, in healthy persons, generally so great that when it has been long resisted, no sensation, however strong it may be, can withstand its power.

Digestion leads to sleep by drawing upon the brain for a portion of its blood. It is for this reason that we feel sleepy after the ingestion of a hearty dinner. A lady of my acquaintance is obliged to sleep a little after each meal. The desire to do so is irresistible; her face becomes pale; her extremities cold; and she sinks into a quiet slumber, which lasts fifteen or twenty minutes. In this lady the amount of blood is not sufficient for the due performance of all the operations of the economy. The digestive organs imperatively require an increased quantity, and the flow takes place from the brain; it being the organ with her which can best spare this fluid. As a rule, persons who eat largely, and have good digestive powers, sleep a great deal, and many persons are unable to sleep at night till they have eaten a substantial supper. The lower animals generally sleep after feeding, especially if the meal has been large.

Excessive loss of blood produces sleep. We can very readily understand why this should be so if we adopt the theory which has been supported in the foregoing pages. It would be exceedingly difficult to explain the fact upon any other hypothesis. I have seen many instances of somnolency due to this cause. It acts not only by directly lessening the quantity of blood in the brain, but also by so enfeebling the heart's action as to prevent a due supply of blood being sent to the cerebral vessels.

Debility is almost always accompanied by a disposition to inordinate sleep. The brain is one of the first organs to feel the effects of a diminished amount of blood or a depraved quality of this fluid being supplied, and hence, in old age, or under the influence of a deficient quantity of food, or through the action of some exhausting disease, there is generally more sleep than when the physical health is not deteriorated.

The action of certain medicines, and of other measures capable of causing sleep, not coming within the range of ordinary application, will be more appropriately considered hereafter.

CHAPTER III.

THE PHYSICAL PHENOMENA OF SLEEP.

THE approach of sleep is characterized by a languor which is agreeable when it can be yielded to, but which, when circumstances prevent this, is far from being pleasant. Many persons are rendered irritable as soon as they become sleepy, and children are especially liable to manifest ill temper under the uncomfortable feelings they experience when unable to indulge the inclination to sleep. It is somewhat difficult to analyze the various phenomena which go to make up the condition called sleepiness. The most prominent feelings are an impression of weight in the upper eyelids, and of a general relaxation of the muscles of the body, but there is besides an internal sensation of supineness, enervation, and torpor, to describe which is by no means easy. This sluggishness is closely allied in character if not altogether identical with that experienced before an attack of fainting, and is doubtless due to a like cause—a deficient quantity of blood in the brain. Along with this languor there is a general obtuseness of all the senses, which increases the separation of the mind from the external world, already initiated by the

(52)

physical condition of the brain. The liveliest scenes cease to engage the attention, and the most exciting conversation no longer interests. For a time, indeed, such circumstances may dissipate the inclination for sleep, but eventually nature obtains the ascendency and consciousness is lost. Before this event there is usually yawning—a phenomenon strongly indicative of a wearied attention; the head nods and droops upon the breast, and the body assumes that position which is most conducive to ease, comfort, and entire muscular inactivity.

The order in which the muscles lose their power is in general well marked, and bears a distinct relation, as Cabanis* has pointed out, to the importance of their functions. Thus, the muscles which move the arms and legs become relaxed before those which support the head, and the latter before those which maintain the erectness of the back. This, however, is not always the case, for, as we have already seen, individuals will occasionally walk, and keep their position on horseback, while in a sound sleep, and all of us have seen persons slumbering in church, their heads dropping on their breasts, but yet firmly holding their prayer-books in their hands under the pretense of going through the services.

As regards the senses, the sight is of course the first to be lost in ordinary cases—the closure of the

---

* Rapports du Physique et du Morale de l'Homme. Paris, 1825, tome ii. p. 381.

eyelids interposing a physical obstruction to the entrance of light. Even when the eyelids have been removed, or from disease cannot be closed, the sight, nevertheless, is the first of the special senses to be abolished. Some animals, as the hare for example, do not shut the eyes when asleep; but even in them the ability to see disappears before the action of the other senses is suspended.

These latter are not altogether abolished during sleep; their acuteness is simply lessened. Taste is the first to fade, and then the smell; hearing follows, and touch yields last of all, and is most readily re-excited. To awake a sleeping person, impressions made upon the sense of touch are more effectual than attempts to arouse through any of the other senses; the hearing comes next in order, smell next, then taste, and the sight is the last of all in capacity for excitation.

During sleep the respiration is slower, deeper, and usually more regular than during wakefulness. The vigor of the process is lessened, and therefore there is a diminution of the pulmonary exhalations. In all probability, also, the ciliated epithelium which lines the air-passages functionates with reduced activity. Owing to this circumstance and to the general muscular torpor which prevails, mucus accumulates in the bronchial tubes and requires to be expectorated on awaking.

The circulation of the blood is rendered slower. The heart beats with more regularity, but with diminished force and frequency. As a consequence the blood is not distributed to distant parts of the body so thoroughly and rapidly as during wakefulness, and accordingly the extremities readily lose their heat. Owing to the reduction in the activity of the respiratory and circulatory functions, the temperature of the whole body falls, and coldness of the atmosphere is less easily resisted.

The functions of the several organs concerned in digestion have their activity increased by sleep. The blood which leaves the brain, goes, as Durham has shown, to the stomach and other abdominal viscera, and hence the quantities of the digestive juices are augmented, and the absorption of the nutritious elements of the food is promoted.

The urine is excreted in less quantity during sleep than when the individual is awake and engaged in mental or physical employment, because the wear and tear of the system is at its minimum.

The perspiration is likewise reduced in amount by sleep. In warm weather, however, the effort to go to sleep often causes an increase in the quantity of this excretion, just as would any other mental or bodily exertion. This circumstance has led some writers to a conclusion the reverse of that just expressed. Others, again, have accepted the doctrine of Sanctorius on this point without stopping to inquire into its correctness. This author,* among

---

* Medicina Statica; or Rules of Health, etc. London, 1676, p. 106 et seq.

other aphorisms relating to sleep, gives the following:

"Undisturbed sleep is so great a promoter of perspiration, that in the space of seven hours, fifty ounces of the concocted perspirable matter do commonly exhale out of strong bodies.

"A man sleeping the space of seven hours is wont, insensibly, healthfully, and without any violence, to perspire twice as much as one awake."

The observations of Sanctorius with his weighing chair led to a good many important results, but they were inexact so far as the function of the skin was concerned, in that they made no division between the loss by this channel and that which takes place through the lungs, for by perspiration in the above quotations he means not only the exhalation from the skin, but the products of respiration—aqueous vapor, carbonic acid, etc. His apparatus was, besides, very imperfect, and could not possibly have given the delicate indications which the subject requires.

Whether the condition of sleep promotes the absorption of morbid growths and accumulations of fluids is very doubtful. Macnish* contends that it does, but *a priori* reasoning would rather lead us to an opposite conclusion. Deficiencies are probably more rapidly made up during sleep than during wakefulness, and thus ulcers heal with more rapidity, owing to the increased formation of granulations

---

Op. cit., p. 6.

which takes place; but the removal of tumors, etc. by natural process involves the operation of forces the very opposite of those concerned in reparation, and observation teaches us that sleep is a condition peculiarly favorable to the deposition of the materials constituting morbid growths. Some writers have alleged that sleep accelerates the absorption of dropsical effusions, but the disappearance of such accumulations during the condition in question is clearly due to the mechanical causes depending upon the position of the body.

It has also been asserted that there is an exaltation of the sexual feeling during sleep. It is difficult to arrive at any very definite conclusion on this point, but it is probable that here again the position of the body conjoined with the heat of the bed has much to do in producing the erotic manifestations occasionally witnessed. Every physician who has had much to do with cases of the kind knows that sleeping upon the back, by which means the blood gravitates to the generative organs and to the lower part of the spinal cord, will often give rise to seminal emissions with or without erotic dreams, and that such occurrences may generally be prevented by the individual avoiding the dorsal decubitus and resting upon one side or the other while asleep. The erections which the generality of healthy men experience in the morning before rising from bed are likewise due to the fact that the recumbent posture favors the flow of blood to the penis and testicles. Such erections are usually unaccompanied by venereal desire.

The ganglionic nervous system and the spinal cord continue in action during sleep, though generally with somewhat diminished power and sensibility. The reflex faculty of the latter organ is still maintained, and thus various movements are executed without the consciousness of the brain being awakened. Somnambulism is clearly a condition of exaltation in the functions of the spinal cord without the controlling influence of the cerebrum being brought into action. But, aside from this rather abnormal phenomenon, there are others which are entirely within the range of health, and which show that the spinal cord is awake, even though the sleep be most profound. Thus, for instance, if the position of the sleeper becomes irksome, it is changed; if the foot become cold, they are drawn up to a warmer part of the bed; and cases are recorded in which individuals have risen from bed and emptied a distended bladder without awaking.

The instances brought forward in a previous chapter of persons riding on horseback and walking during sleep show the activity of the spinal cord, and not that the will is exercised; and Cabanis* is wrong in the view which he gives of such phenomena in the following extract.

Speaking of cases like those just referred to, he says:

---

* Op. cit., tome ii. p. 385.

"These rare instances are not the only ones in which movements are observed produced during sleep by that portion of the will which is awake; for it is by virtue of certain direct sensations that a sleeping man moves his arm to brush away the flies from his face, that he draws the cover around him so as to envelop himself carefully, or that he turns in bed till he has found a comfortable position. It is the will which during sleep maintains the contraction of the sphincter of the bladder, notwithstanding the effort of the urine to escape."

Such examples as the above we now know to be instances of reflex action, and as not, therefore, being due to the exercise of the will.

Sleep favors the occurrence of certain pathological phenomena. Thus individuals affected with hæmorrhoids have the liability to hemorrhage increased when they are asleep. Several instances of the kind have come under my notice. In one the patient lost so large a quantity of blood that syncope ensued and might have terminated fatally had not his condition been accidentally discovered. Bleeding from the lungs is also more apt to occur during sleep in those who are predisposed to it. Darwin states that a man of about fifty years of age, subject to hæmorrhoids, was also attacked with hæmoptysis three consecutive nights at about the same hour—two o'clock —being awakened thereby from a state of very profound sleep. He was advised to suffer himself to be roused at one o'clock, and to leave his bed at that hour. He did so with the result not only of entirely breaking up the hemorrhagic disposition, but also of curing himself of very violent attacks of headache, to which he had been subject for many years.

Epileptic fits are also more liable to occur during sleep than at other times, a fact not always susceptible of easy explanation. In a case of epilepsy now under my charge, this proclivity is so well marked that the patient, a lady, scarcely ever goes to sleep without being attacked. Her face becomes exceedingly pale just before the fit, and if then seen the paroxysm can be entirely prevented by waking her. She is never attacked at other times, and I am trying, with excellent results thus far, the plan of making her sleep altogether during the day and of waking her as soon as her face becomes pallid. It is probable that the fits in her case are due to a diminished amount of blood in the brain, and this supposition is strengthened by the additional fact that bromide of potassium—a substance which, as I have shown, lessens the amount of intracranial blood—invariably rendered her paroxysms more frequent and severe.

Sleep predisposes to attacks of gout in those who have the gouty diathesis, and likewise favors exacerbations in several other diseases which it is scarcely necessary to allude to specifically. The accession of fever toward night, and the increase which takes place in pain due to inflammation are generally associated with the approach of night, and have no direct relation with sleep.

Certain other morbid phenomena, such as somnambulism and nightmare, which have a necessary
relation with sleep, will be more appropriately considered in another place.

On the other hand, sleep controls the manifestations of several diseases, especially those which are
of a convulsive or spasmodic character. Thus the
paroxysms of chorea cease during sleep, as do likewise the spasms of tetanus and hydrophobia. Headache is also generally relieved by sleep, though
occasionally it is aggravated.

6

CHAPTER IV.

THE STATE OF THE MIND DURING SLEEP.

WE have seen that though during sleep the operations of the senses are entirely suspended as regards the effects of ordinary impressions, the purely animal functions of the body continue in action. The heart beats, the lungs respire, the stomach, the intestines, and their accessory organs digest, the skin exhales vapor, and the kidneys secrete urine. With the central nervous system, however, the case is very different; for while some parts retain the property of receiving impressions or developing ideas, others have their actions diminished, exalted, perverted, or altogether arrested.

In the first place, there is, undoubtedly, during sleep, a general torpor of the sensorium, which prevents the appreciation of the ordinary excitations made upon the organs of the special senses. So far as the nerves themselves are concerned, there is no loss of their irritability or conducting power, and the impressions made upon them are, accordingly, perfectly well conveyed to the brain. The suspension of the operations of the senses is not therefore due to any loss of function in the optic nerve, the

(62)

auditory nerve, the olfactory nerve, the gustatorv nerve, or the cranial or spinal nerves concerned in the sense of touch, but solely to the inability of the brain to take cognizance of the impressions conveyed to it. In regard to the cause of this torpor, I have given my views in a previous chapter.

Now it must not be supposed that because mild excitations transmitted by the nerves of the special senses are incapable of making themselves felt, that therefore the brain is in a state of complete repose throughout all its parts. So far from such a condition existing, there are very decided proofs that several faculties are exercised to a degree almost equaling that reached during wakefulness, and we know that if the irritations made upon the senses be sufficiently strong, the brain *does* appreciate them, and the sleep is broken. This ability to be readily roused through the senses constitutes one of the main differences between sleep and stupor, upon which stress has been already laid.

Relative to the different faculties of the mind. as affected by sleep, great variations are observed. It has been thought by some authors that several of them are really exalted above the standard attained during wakefulness, but this is probably a wrong view. The predominance which one or two mental qualities apparently assume is not due to any absolute exaggeration of power, but to the suspension of the action of other faculties, which, when we are not asleep, exercise a governing or modifying influence.

Thus, for instance, as regards the imagination,—the
faculty of all others which appears to be most increased,—we find, when we carefully study its manifestations in our own persons, that although there is
often great brilliancy in its vagaries, that uncon-
trolled as it is by the judgment, the pictures which
it paints upon our minds are usually incongruous
and silly in the extreme.   Even though the train of
ideas excited by this faculty when we are asleep be
rational and coherent, we are fully conscious on
awaking that we are capable of doing much better
by intentionally setting the brain in action and governing it by our will and judgment.

Owing to the fact that these two faculties of the
mind are incapable of acting normally during sleep,
the imagination is left absolutely without controlling
influence.   Indeed, we are often cognizant in those
dreams which take place when we are half awake,
of an inability to direct it.   The impressions which
it makes upon the mind are, therefore, intense, but
of very little durability.   Many stories are told of
its power—how problems have been worked out,
poetry and music composed, and great undertakings
planned; but if we could get at the truth, we should
probably find that the imagination of sleep had very
little to do with the operations mentioned.   Indeed,
it is doubtful if the mind of a sleeping person can
originate ideas.   Those which are formed are, as
Locke* remarks, almost invariably made up of the

---

* An Essay concerning Human Understanding.   Book ii. sect. 17

waking man's ideas, and are for the most part very oddly put together; and we are all aware how commonly our dreams are composed of ideas, or based upon events which have recently occurred to us.

In the previous section to the one just quoted, Locke refers to the exaggeration of ideas which form so common a feature of our mental actions during sleep. "It is true," he says, "we have sometimes instances of perception while we are asleep, and retain the memory of those thoughts; but how extravagant and incoherent for the most part they are, how little conformable to the perfection and order of a rational being, those acquainted with dreams need not be told."

And yet many remarkable stories are related, which tend to show the high degree of activity possessed by the mind during sleep. Thus it is said of Tartini,* a celebrated musician of the eighteenth century, that one night he dreamed he had made a compact with the devil, and bound him to his service. In order to ascertain the musical abilities of his servitor, he gave him his violin, and commanded him to play a solo. The devil did so, and performed so admirably that Tartini awoke with the excitement produced, and seizing his violin, endeavored to repeat

---

* Encyclopedia Americana,—Philadelphia, 1832, vol. xii. p. 143, art. Tartini; and L'Imagination considérée dans ses Effets directs sur l'Homme et les Animaux, etc. Par J. B. Demangeon. Seconde édition. Paris, 1829, p. 161.

the enchanting air. Although he was unable to do this with entire success, his efforts were so far effectual that he composed one of the most admired of his pieces, which in recognition of its source he called the "devil's sonata."

Coleridge gives the following account of the composition of the fragment, Kubla Khan·

"In the summer of 1797, the author, then in ill health, had retired to a lonely farm-house, between Perlock and Linton, on the Exmoor confines of Somerset and Devonshire In consequence of a slight indisposition, an anodyne had been prescribed, from the effects of which he fell asleep in his chair at the moment that he was reading the following sentence, or words of the same substance, in Purchas's Pilgrimage: 'Here the Khan Kubla commanded a palace to be built, and a stately garden thereunto. And thus ten miles of fertile ground were inclosed with a wall.' The author continued for about three hours in a profound sleep, at least of the external senses, during which time he had the most vivid confidence that he could have composed not less than from two to three hundred lines, if that, indeed, can be called composition, in which all the images rose up before him as *things* with a parallel production of the corresponding expression without any sensation or consciousness of effort. On awaking, he appeared to himself to have a distinct recollection of the whole; and taking his pen, ink, and paper, instantly and eagerly wrote down the lines that are here preserved. At this moment he was unfortunately called out by a person on business from Perlock, and detained by him above an hour; and on his return to his room, found to his no small surprise and mortification, that though he still retained some vague and dim recollection of the general purport of the vision, yet with the exception of some eight or ten scattered lines and images, all the rest had passed away like the images on the surface of a stream into which a stone had been cast, but, alas! without the after restoration of the latter."

Dr. Cromwell,* citing the above instance of poetic inspiration during sleep, states that, having like Coleridge taken an anodyne during a painful illness, he composed the following lines of poetry, which he wrote down within half an hour after awaking. These lines, though displaying considerable imagination, are not remarkable for any other quality.

"Lines composed in sleep on the night of January 9th, 1857.

" SCENE.— *Windsor Forest.*

"At a vista's end stood the queen one day
Relieved by a sky of the softest hue;
It happen'd that a wood-mist risen new,
Had made that white which should have been blue.
A sunbeam sought on her form to play;

---

* The Soul and the Future Life. Appendix viii. Quoted by Seafield in "The Literature and Curiosities of Dreams," etc. London, 1865. Vol. ii. p. 229.

It found a nook in the bowery nave,
Through which with its golden stem to lave
And kiss the leaves of the stately trees
That fluttered and rustled beneath the breeze;
But it touched not her, to whom 'twas given
To walk in a white light pure as heaven."

In the last two of these instances it is impossible
to say whether the individuals were really asleep or
not, as the opium or other narcotic taken is a very
disturbing factor in both conditions, and doubtless
was the exciting cause of the activity in the imagination.   No more graphic account of the effects of
opium in arousing the imagination to its highest
pitch has been written than that given by De Quincey.*   He says:
"At night when I lay awake in bed, vast processions passed along in mournful pomp; friezes of
never-ending stories, that to my feelings were as sad
and solemn as if they were stories drawn from times
before Œdipus or Priam, before Tyre, before Mem-
phis.   And at the same time a corresponding change
took place in my dreams; a theater seemed suddenly
opened and lighted up within my brain, which presented nightly spectacles of more than earthly splen-
dor."   And then, after referring to the various scenes
of architectural magnificence, and of beautiful women which his imagination conceived, and which
forcibly recalls to our minds the poetical effusions

* Confessions of an English Opium-eater.   Boston, 1866, p. 109.

of Coleridge and Cromwell, he gives the details of another dream, in which he heard music. "A music of preparation, of awakening suspense; a music like the opening of the Coronation Anthem, and which like *that* gave the feeling of a vast march, of infinite cavalcades filing off, and the tread of innumerable armies."

In reference to this subject, Dr. Forbes Winslow* relates the following interesting case:

"A feeble, sensitive lady, suffering from a uterine affection, writes to us as follows concerning the influence of three or four sixteenth-of-a-grain doses of hydrochlorate of morphia: 'After taking a few doses of morphia, I felt a sensation of extreme quiet and wish for repose, and on closing my eyes, visions, if I may so call them, were constantly before me, and as constantly changing in their aspect: scenes from foreign lands; lovely landscapes, with tall, magnificent trees covered with drooping foliage, which was blown gently against me as I walked along. Then in an instant I was in a besieged city filled with armed men. I was carrying an infant, which was snatched from me by a soldier and killed upon the spot. A Turk was standing by with a scimitar in his hand, which I seized, and attacking the man who had killed the child, I fought most furiously with him and killed him. Then I was surrounded, made

---

* Journal of Psychological Medicine and Mental Pathology. July, 1859, p. 44.

prisoner, carried before a judge and accused of the deed; but I pleaded my own cause with such a burst of eloquence (which, by-the-by, I am quite incapable of in my right mind) that judge, jury, and hearers acquitted me at once. Again, I was in an Eastern city visiting an Oriental lady, who entertained me most charmingly. We sat together on rich ottomans, and were regaled with supper and confectionery. Then came soft sounds of music at a distance, while fountains were playing and birds singing, and dancing girls danced before us, every movement being accompanied with the tinkling of silver bells attached to their feet. But all this suddenly changed, and I was entertaining the Oriental lady in my own house, and in order to please her delicate taste, I had everything prepared as nearly as possible after the fashion with which she had so enchanted me. She, however, to my no small surprise, asked for wine, and took not one, two, or three glasses, but drank freely, until at last I became terrified that she would have to be carried away intoxicated. While considering what course I had better adopt, several English officers came in, and she at once asked them to drink with her, which so shocked my sense of propriety that the scene changed and I was in darkness.

" 'Then I felt that I was formed of granite, and immovable. Suddenly a change came again over me, and I found that I consisted of delicate and fragile basket-work. Then I became a danseuse, delighting an audience and myself by movements which seemed barely to touch the earth. Presently beautiful sights came before me, treasures from the depth of the sea, gems of the brightest hues, gorgeous shells, coral of the richest colors, sparkling with drops of water, and hung with lovely seaweed. My eager glances could not take in half the beautiful objects that passed before me during the inecssant changes the visions underwent. Now I was gazing upon antique brooches and rings from buried cities; now upon a series of Egyptian vases; now upon sculptured wood-work blackened by time; and lastly I was buried amid forests of tall trees, such as I had read of but never seen.

"'The sights that pleased me most I had power to a certain extent to prolong, and those that displeased me I could occasionally set aside, and I awoke myself to full consciousness once or twice while under the influence of the morphia by an angry exclamation that I would not have it. I did not once lose my personal identity.'

"The lady almost invariably suffers more or less from hallucinations of the foregoing character, if it becomes necessary to administer to her an opiate: and on analyzing her visions, she can generally refer the principal portions of them, notwithstanding their confusion and distortion, to works that she has recently read."

Opium, in certain doses, increases the amount of blood in the brain, and this induces a condition very

different from that of sleep.   In this fact we have
an explanation of the activity of the imagination as
one of its prominent effects.   That Coleridge should
have composed the Kubla Khan under its influence
is in nowise remarkable.   It is probable, however,
that the full influence of his mind was exerted upon
it after he awoke to consciousness, and that the wild
fancies excited by the opiate, and based upon what
he had been previously reading, formed the sub-
stratum of his conceptions.   In any event, the ideas
contained in this fragment are no more fanciful than
those which occurred to De Quincey and the lady
whose case has just been recorded, nor are they
more impressively related.

The imagination may therefore be active during
sleep, but we have no authentic instance on record
that it has, unaided by causes which exercise a powerful influence over the intracranial circulation, led
to the production of any ideas which could not be
excelled by the individual when awake.   Perhaps
the most striking case in opposition to this opinion
is one detailed by Abercrombie,* who says:

" The following anecdote has been preserved in a
family of rank in Scotland, the descendants of a
distinguished lawyer of the last age.   This eminent
person had been consulted respecting a case of great
importance and much difficulty, and he had been
studying it with intense anxiety and attention.

* Inquiries concerning the Intellectual Powers and the Investigation of Truth.   Tenth edition.   London, 1840, p. 304.

After several days had been occupied in this manner, he was observed by his wife to rise from his bed in the night and go to a writing-desk which stood in the bed-room. He then sat down and wrote a long letter, which he put carefully by in the desk and returned to bed. The following morning he told his wife that be had had a most interesting dream; that he had dreamt of delivering a clear and luminous opinion respecting a case which had exceedingly perplexed him, and that he would give anything to recover the train of thought which had passed before him in his dream. She then directed him to the writing-desk, where he found the opinion clearly and fully written out, and which was afterwards found to be perfectly correct."

It is probable that this gentleman was actually awake when he arose from the bed and wrote the paper referred to, and that in the morning he mistook the circumstance for a dream. It is not at all uncommon for such errors to be committed, especially under the condition of mental anxiety and fatigue. A gentleman informed me only a short time since that going to bed after a very exciting day he thought the next morning that he had dreamed of a fire occurring in the vicinity of his house. To his surprise his wife informed him that the supposed dream was a reality, and that he had got up to the window, looked at the fire, conversed with her concerning it, and that he was at the time fully awake.

Brierre de Boismont* relates the following instance, which is to the same effect:

"In a convent in Auvergne, an apothecary was sleeping with several persons; being attacked with nightmare, he charged his companions with throwing themselves on him and attempting to strangle him. They all denied the assertion, telling him that he had passed the night without sleeping, and in a state of high excitement. In order to convince him of this fact, they prevailed on him to sleep alone in a room carefully closed, having previously given him a good supper, and even made him partake of food of a flatulent nature. The paroxysm returned; but, on this occasion, he swore that it was the work of a demon, whose face and figure he perfectly described."

That the imagination may in its flights during sleep strike upon fancies which are subsequently developed by the reason into lucid and valuable ideas, is very probable. It would be strange if from among the innumerable absurdities and extravagancies to which it attains something fit to be appropriated by the mind should not occasionally be evolved, and thus there are many instances mentioned of the starting-point of important mental operations having been taken during sleep. Some of these may be based upon fact, but the majority are probably of

---

* A History of Dreams, Visions, Apparitions, etc. Philadelphia, 1855, p. 184.

the class of those just specified, or occurred at an age of the world when a belief in the supernatural exercised a greater power over men's minds than it does at the present day. Among the most striking of them are the following:

Galen declares that he owed a great part of his knowledge to the revelations made to him in dreams. Whether this was really the case or not we can in a measure determine by recalling the fact that he was a believer in the prophetic nature of dreams, and states that a man having dreamt that one of his legs was turned into stone, soon afterward became paralytic in this limb, although there was no evidence of approaching disease. Galen also conducted his practice by dreams, for an athlete, having dreamt that he saw red spots, and that the blood was flowing out of his body, was supposed by Galen to require blood-letting, which operation was accordingly performed.

It has been said* that the idea of the *Divina Commedia* occurred to Dante during sleep. There is nothing at all improbable in this supposition, though I have been unable to trace it to any definite source.

Cabanis† states that Condillac assured him that often during the course of his studies he had to leave them unfinished in order to sleep, and that on

---

* Macario, Du Sommeil, des Rêves et du Somnambulisme. Paris, 1857, p. 59.

† Op. cit., tome ii. p. 395.

awaking he had more than once found the work upon which he was engaged brought to a conclusion in his brain.

These were clearly instances of "unconscious cerebration" of that power which the brain possesses to work out matters which have engaged its attention, without the consciousness of the individual being aroused to a knowledge of the labor being performed. It is not unlikely that this kind of mental activity goes on to some extent during sleep, but as it is of such a character that the mind does not take cognizance of its operations, I do not see how the exact period of its performance can be ascertained.

Jerome Cardan believed that he composed books while asleep, and his case is often adduced as an example of the height to which the imagination can attain during sleep. But this great man was superstitious to an extreme degree; he believed that he had a familiar spirit, from whom he received intelligence, warnings, and ideas, and asserted that when awake he frequently saw long processions of men, women, animals, trees, castles, instruments of various kinds and many figures, different from anything in this world. His evidence relative to his compositions and mathematical labors when asleep is not therefore of a trustworthy character.

As regards the memory in sleep, it is undoubtedly exercised to a considerable extent. In fact, whatever degree of activity the mind may then exhibit is based upon events the recollection of which has been retained.   But there is more or less error mingled with a small amount of truth.   The un-bridled imagination of the sleeper so distorts the simplest circumstances as to render their recognition a matter of no small difficulty, and thus it scarcely if ever happens that events are reproduced during sleep exactly as they occurred or as they would be recalled by the mind of the individual when awake. Frequently, also, recent events which have made a strong impression on our minds are forgotten, as when we dream of seeing and conversing with per-sons not long dead.

And yet it has sometimes happened that incidents or knowledge which had long been overlooked or forgotten, or which could not be remembered by any effort during wakefulness have been strongly depicted during sleep.   Thus Lord Monboddo* states that the Countess de Laval, a woman of per-feet veracity and good sense, when ill, spoke during sleep in a language which none of her attendants understood, and which even she was disposed to re-gard as gibberish.   A nurse detected the dialect of Brittany; her mistress had spent her childhood in that province, but had lost all recollection of the Breton tongue, and could not understand a word of what she said in her dreams.   Her utterances ap-

---

* Ancient Metaphysics.   Quoted in Dr. Forbes Winslow's Medi-cal Critic and Psychological Journal.   No. vi., April, 1862, p. 206.

plied, however, exclusively to the experience of childhood, and were infantile in structure.

Abercrombie* relates the case of a gentleman who was very fond of the Greek language, and who, in his youth, had made considerable progress in it. Subsequently being engaged in other pursuits, he so entirely forgot it that he could not even read the words; often, however, in his dreams he read Greek works, which he had been accustomed to use at college, and had a most vivid impression of fully understanding them.

Many other instances of the action of memory during sleep might be brought forward, but the subject will be more appropriately considered in the chapter on dreams.

The judgment is frequently exercised when we are asleep, but almost invariably in a perverted manner. In fact we scarcely ever estimate the events or circumstances which appear to transpire in our dreams at their real value, and very rarely from correct conceptions of right and wrong. High-minded and honorable men do not scruple during sleep to sanction the most atrocious acts, or to regard with complaisance ideas which, in their waking moments, would fill them with horror. Delicate and refined women will coolly enter upon a career of crime, and the minds of hardened villains are filled with the most elevated and noble

---

* Op. cit., p. 283.

sentiments. The deeds which we imagine we perform in our sleep are generally inadequate to or in excess of what the apparent occasion requires, and we lose so entirely the ideas of probability and possibility, that no preposterous vision appears otherwise than as perfectly natural and correct. Thus, a physician dreamed that he had been transformed into a monolith which stood grandly and alone in the vast desert of the Sahara, and had so stood for ages, while generation after generation wasted and melted away around him. Although unconscious of having organs of sense, this column of granite saw the mountains growing bald with age, the forests drooping with decay, and the moss and ivy creeping around its crumbling base.*

But, although in this instance there was some conception of time, as shown in the association of the evidences of decay with the lapse of years, there is in general no correct idea on this subject. Without going into details which more appropriately belong to another division of this treatise, I quote the following remarkable example from the essay last cited. It appeared originally in a biographical sketch of Lavalette, published in the *Revue de Paris*, and is related by Lavalette as occurring to him while in prison:

"One night, while I was asleep, the clock of the

* Dream Thought and Dream Life. Medical Critic and Psychological Journal, No. vi., April, 1862, p. 199.

Palais de Justice struck twelve and awoke me. I heard the gate open to relieve the sentry, but I fell asleep again immediately. In this sleep I dreamt that I was standing in the Rue St. Honore. A melancholy darkness spread around me; all was still; nevertheless, a slow and uncertain sound soon arose. All of a sudden, I perceived at the bottom of the street and advancing toward me, a troop of cavalry,—the men and horses, however, all flayed. The men held torches in their hands, the red flames of which illuminated faces without skin, and bloody muscles. Their hollow eyes rolled fearfully in their sockets, their mouths opened from ear to ear, and helmets of hanging flesh covered their hideous heads. The horses dragged along their own skins in the kennels which overflowed with blood on all sides. Pale and disheveled women appeared and disappeared at the windows in dismal silence; low inarticulate groans filled the air, and I remained in the street alone petrified with horror, and deprived of strength sufficient to seek my safety in flight. This horrible troop continued passing along rapidly in a gallop, and casting frightful looks upon me. Their march continued, I thought, for five hours, and they were followed by an immense number of artillery wagons full of bleeding corpses, whose limbs still quivered; a disgusting smell of blood and bitumen almost choked me. At length the iron gates of the prison, shutting with great force, awoke me again. I made my repeater strike; it was no more than midnight, so that the horrible phantasmagoria had lasted no more than two or three minutes—that is to say, the time necessary for relieving the sentry and shutting the gate. The cold was severe and the watchword short. The next day the turnkey confirmed my calculations. I, nevertheless, do not remember one single event in my life the duration of which I have been able more exactly to calculate, of which the details are deeper engraven on my memory, and of which I preserve a more perfect consciousness."

No instance can more strikingly exemplify aberration of the faculty of judgment than the above. There was no astonishment felt with the horror experienced, but all the impossible events which appeared to be transpiring were accepted as facts which might have taken place in the regular order of nature.

An important question connected with the exercise of judgment is: does the dreamer know that he is dreaming? Some authors assert that this knowledge is possible, others that it is not. The following account is interesting, and I therefore transcribe it, especially as it has not to my knowledge been heretofore published in this country.

In a letter to the Rev. William Gregory, Dr. Thomas Reid* says:

---

* Account of the Life and Writings of Thomas Reid, D.D , p. cxliv., prefixed to Essays on the Powers of the Human Mind. By Thomas Reid, **D.D** , etc. Edinburgh, 1803, vol. i.

"About the age of fourteen, I was almost every night unhappy in my sleep from frightful dreams. Sometimes hanging over a frightful precipice and just ready to drop down; sometimes pursued for my life and stopped by a wall or by a sudden loss of all strength; sometimes ready to be devoured by a wild beast. How long I was plagued by such dreams I do not now recollect. I believe it was for a year or two at least; and I think they had quite left me before I was fifteen. In those days I was much given to what Mr. Addison in one of his Spectators calls castle-building, and, in my evening solitary walk, which was generally all the exercise I took, my thoughts would hurry me into some active scene, where I generally acquitted myself much to my own satisfaction, and in these scenes of imagination I performed many a gallant exploit. At the same time, in my dreams, I found myself the most arrant coward that ever was. Not only my courage, but my strength failed me in every danger, and I often rose from my bed in the morning in such a panic that it took some time to get the better of it. I wished very much to get free of these uneasy dreams, which not only made me unhappy in sleep, but often left a disagreeable impression in my mind for some part of the following day. I thought it was worth trying whether it was possible to recollect that it was all a dream, and that I was in no real danger. I often went to sleep with my mind as strongly impressed as I could with this thought that I never in my lifetime was in any real danger, and that every fright I had was a dream. After many fruitless endeavors to recollect this when the danger appeared, I effected it at last, and have often, when I was sliding over a precipice into the abyss, recollected that it was all a dream, and boldly jumped down. The effect of this commonly was, that I immediately awoke. But I awoke calm and intrepid, which I thought a great acquisition. After this my dreams were never very uneasy, and, in a short time, I dreamed not at all."

Beattie[*] states that he once dreamed that he was walking on the parapet of a high bridge. How he came there he did not know, but recollecting that he was not given to such pranks, he began to think it might all be a dream, and, finding his situation unpleasant, and being desirous to get out of it, threw himself headlong from the height, in the belief that the shock of the fall would restore his senses. The event turned out as he anticipated.

Aristotle also asserts that when dreaming of danger, he used to recollect that he was dreaming, and that he ought not to be frightened.

A still more remarkable narration is that of Gassendi,[†] which he thus relates as occurring to himself:

---

[*] Dissertations, Moral and Critical. London, 1783, art. Dreaming, p. 222.

[†] Syntagma Philosophicum. Pars 71, Lib. viii. Opera Omnia, tome i. Lugduni, 1658.

"A good friend of mine, Louis Charambon, judge of the criminal court at Digne, had died of the plague. One night, as I slept, I seemed to see him; I stretched out my arms toward him, and said, 'Hail thou who returnest from the place of the dead!' Then I stopped, reflecting in my dream as follows: 'One cannot return from the other world; I am doubtless dreaming; but if I dream, where am I? Not at Paris, for I came last to Digne. I am then at Digne, in my house, in my bedroom, in my bed.' And then, as I was looking for myself in the bed, some noise, I know not what, awoke me."

In all these and like instances, it is very probable the individuals were much more awake than asleep, for certainly the power to judge correctly is not exercised in dreams, involving even the most incongruous impossibilities. As Dendy* says, "if we *know* that we are dreaming, the faculty of judgment cannot be inert, and the dream would be known to be a fallacy." There would therefore be no occasion for any such management of it as that made use of by Reid and Beattie, or for the recollection of Aristotle. The dream and the correction of it by the judgment would go together and there would be no self-deception at all—not even for an instant. Dreams would accordingly be impossible. The essential feature of mental activity during sleep, absolute freedom of the imagination, would not exist.

---

* Philosophy of Mystery. London, 1841, p. 208.

Relative to Gassendi's case, it is impossible to believe that he was fully asleep, and the fact that he was awakened by some noise, the nature of which was unrecognized, and which was therefore probably slight, tends to support this view. Moreover, although he was, as he thought, enabled to detect the fallacy of his dream in one respect, his judgment was altogether at fault in others. Thus he had great difficulty in making out where he was, and actually so far lost all idea of his identity with the person dreaming as to look for himself in his own bed! Certainly an individual whose judgment was thus much deranged would scarcely be able to reason correctly as to the fact of his dreaming or not, or to question the possibility of the dead returning to this world.

My opinion therefore is, that during sleep the power of bringing the judgment into action is suspended. We do not actually lose the power of arriving at a decision, but we cannot exert the faculty of judgment in accordance with the principles of truth and of correct reasoning. An opinion may therefore be formed during sleep, but it is more likely to be wrong than right, and no effort that we can make will enable us to distinguish the false from the true, or to discriminate between the possible and the impossible.

That faculty of the mind—the judgment—which when we are awake is pre-eminently our guide, can no longer direct us aright. The stores of experience go for naught, and the mind accepts as truth whatever preposterous thought the imagination presents to it. We are not entirely rendered incapable of judging, as some authors assert, but the power to perceive the logical force of circumstances, to take them at their true value and to eliminate error from our mental processes, is altogether arrested, and we arrive at absurd conclusions from impossible premises.

But there is no doubt that at times the faculty of judgment is suspended as regards some parts of our mental operations during sleep, and this, to such an extent, that we are like Gassendi in the case quoted, not capable of recognizing our own individuality. Thus it is related of Dr. Johnson, that he had once in a dream a contest of wit with some other person, and that he was very much mortified by imagining that his opponent had the better of him "Now," said he, "one may mark here the effect of sleep in weakening the power of reflection; for had not my judgment failed me, I should have seen that the wit of this supposed antagonist, by whose superiority I felt myself depressed, was as much furnished by me as that which I thought I had been uttering in mv own character."

Van Goens dreamt that he could not answer questions to which his neighbor gave correct responses.

An interesting case, in which the judgment was still more at fault, has recently come to my knowledge.

Mrs. C. dreamed that she was Savonarola, and that she was preaching to a vast assembly in Florence. Among the audience was a lady whom she at once recognized to be her own self. As Savonarola, she was delighted at this discovery, for she reflected that she was well acquainted with all Mrs. C.'s peculiarities and faults of character, and would, therefore, be enabled to give special emphasis to them in the sermon. She did this so very effectively that Mrs. C. burst into a torrent of tears, and, with the emotion thus excited, the lady awoke. It was some time before she was able to disentangle her mixed up individualities. When she became fully awake she perceived that the arguments she had employed to bring about the conversion of herself were puerile in the extreme, and were directed against characteristics which formed no part of her mental organization, and against offenses which she had not committed.

Macario* makes the following apposite remarks on the point under consideration. Referring to the preposterous nature of many dreams, he says:

"It is astonishing that all these fantastical and impossible visions seem to us quite natural, and excite no astonishment. This is because the judgment and reflection having abdicated, no longer control the imagination nor co-ordinate the thoughts which rush tumultuously through the brain of the sleeper, combined only by the power of association.

---

* Op. cit., p. 286.

"When I say that the judgment and reflection abdicate, it should not be inferred that they are abolished and no longer exist, for the imagination could not, unaided by the reason, construct the whimsical and capricious images of dreams."

Relative to the power to work out, during sleep, problems involving long and intricate mental processes, I have already expressed my opinion adversely. In this view, I am not alone. Rosenkranz,* whose contributions to psychological science cannot be overestimated, and whose clear and powerful understanding has rarely been excelled, has pointed out how such operations of the understanding are impossible; for, as he remarks, intellectual problems cannot be solved during sleep, for such a thing as intense thought, accompanied by images, is unknown, whilst dreams consist of a series of images connected by loose and imperfect reasoning. Feuchtersleben,† referring with approval to this opinion of Rosenkranz, says that he recollects perfectly having dreamt of such problems, and being happy in their solution, endeavored to retain them in his memory; he succeeded, but discovered, on awaking, that they were quite unmeaning, and could only have imposed upon a sleeping imagination.

---

* Psychologie; oder der Wissenschaft von Subjectiven Geist. 2ten Auflage. Ebberfeld, 1843, p. 144.

† The Principles of Medical Psychology, etc. Sydenham Society Translation, p 167.

Müller* says:

"Sometimes we reason more or less correctly in dreams. We reflect on problems and rejoice in their solution. But on awaking from such dreams, the seeming reasoning is frequently found to have been no reasoning at all, and the solution of the problem over which we had rejoiced, to be mere nonsense. Sometimes we dream that another person proposes an enigma; that we cannot solve it and that others are equally incapable of doing so; but that the person who proposed it, himself gives the explanation. We are astonished at the solution we had so long labored in vain to find. If we do not immediately awaken and afterwards reflect on this proposition of an enigma in our dream, and on its apparent solution, we think it wonderful; but if we awake immediately after the dream, and are able to compare the answer with the question, we find that it was mere nonsense."

And in regard to the knowledge that we are dreaming, the same author† observes that:

"The indistinctness of the conception in dreams is generally so great that we are not aware that we dream. The phantasms which are perceived really exist in our organs of sense. They afford, there- fore, in themselves as strong proof of the actual ex-

---

* Elements of Physiology. Translated from the German, with Notes, by William Baly, M D., etc.   London, 1842, vol. ii. p. 1417.

† Op. cit., p. 1418.

istence of the objects they represent, as our own
perceptions of real external objects in the waking
state ; for we know the latter only by the affections
of our senses which they produce.   When, therefore, the mind has lost the faculty of analyzing
the impressions on our senses, there is no reason
why the things which they seem to represent should
be supposed unreal.   Even in the waking state
phantasms are regarded as real objects when they
occur to persons of feeble intellect.   On the other
hand, when the dreaming approaches more nearly
to the waking state, we sometimes are conscious
that we merely dream, and still allow the dream to
proceed, while we retain this consciousness of its
true nature.''

Sir Benjamin Brodie,* in discussing the subject
of wonderful discoveries made in dreams, and abstruse problems worked out, remarks that it would
indeed be strange if among the vast number of com-
binations which constitute our dreams, there were
not every now and then some having the semblance
of reality; and further, that in many of the stories
of great discoveries made in dreams, there is much
of either mistake or exaggeration, and that if they
could have been written down at the time, they
would have been found to be worth little or nothing.

Another faculty exercised during sleep has been

* Psychological Inquiries. Part i. London, 1856, p. 153.

ascribed to the judgment. It is well known that many persons having made up their minds to awake at a certain hour invariably do so. I possess this power in a high degree, and scarcely ever vary a minute from the fixed time. Just as I go to bed I look at my watch and impress upon my mind the figures on the dial which represent the hour and minute at which I wish to awake. I give myself no further anxiety on the subject, and never dream of it, but I always wake at the desired moment.

Now I cannot conceive what connection the judgment has with this power. In the ease of alarm clocks set to go off at a certain time, the judgment, as Jouffroy* asserts, may take cognizance of the impression made upon the ear, and establish the relation between it and the wish to awake at a certain time. But in cases where the awaking is the result of an idea conceived before going to sleep, and which is not subsequently recalled, the judgment cannot act, for this faculty is only exercised upon ideas which are submitted to it. The brain is, as it were, wound up like the alarm clock and set to a certain hour. When that hour arrives, an explosion of nervous force takes place, and the individual awakes.

Fosgate† asserts that the power of judging during sleep is probably as good as when we are awake, for

---

* Du Sommeil—Mélanges Philosophiques. Seconde édition. Paris, 1838, p. 301.

† Sleep Psychologically considered with reference to Sensation and Memory. New York, 1850, p. 74.

decisions are made only on the premises presented in either case, and if those in the former condition are absurd or unreasonable, the conclusion will likewise be faulty. But this is not very accurate reasoning; for it is as much the province of the judgment to determine the validity of the premises as it is to draw a conclusion from them, and if it cannot recognize the falsity or truth of propositions the irrational character of which would be readily perceived during wakefulness, there is not much to be said in favor of its power.

In fact, however, the conclusions formed in dreams are often without any logical relation with the premises. Thus, when an individual dreams, as in the instance previously quoted, that he is a column of stone, it is contrary to all experience to deduce therefrom the conclusion that he can see rocks crumbling around him, and can reflect upon the mutability of all things. The premise of his being a stone pillar being submitted to the judgment, the proper conclusion would be that he is composed of inorganic material, is devoid of life, and consequently not possessed of either sensation or understanding.

Why the judgment is not properly exercised during sleep we do not know. Dr. Philip* believes that in this condition ideas flow so rapidly that they

---

* An Inquiry into the Nature of Sleep and Death. London, 1834, p. 152. (Reprinted from the Philosophical Transactions for 1833.)

are not submitted to the full power of the judgment, and that hence the absurdity which characterizes them is not perceived. But this explanation is by no means satisfactory; for a merely swift succession of ideas is no very serious bar to correct judgment, and when the thoughts are as preposterous as those which so often occur in dreams, they present no obstacle at all to a proper estimation of them by the healthy mind. The cause probably resides in some alteration in the circulation of the blood in that part of the brain which presides over the judgment, whereby its power is suspended and the imagination left free to fill the mind with its incongruous and fantastic images.

As regards the will, we find very opposite opinions entertained relative to its activity; but no one, so far as I am aware, appears to have had correct views upon the subject. Without going into a full discussion of the views enunciated, it will be sufficient to refer to the ideas on the point in question which have been expressed by some of the most eminent philosophers and physiologists.

In the course of his remarks on sleep, Darwin* repeatedly alleges that during this condition the action of the will is entirely suspended; but he falls into the singular error of confounding volition with the power of motion. Thus he says:

---

* Zoonomia; or, The Laws of Organic Life. Am. ed , vol. i. Philadelphia, 1818, p. 153.

"When by one continued posture in sleep some uneasy sensations are produced, we either gradually awake by the exertion of volition, or the muscles connected by habit with such sensations alter the position of the body; but where the sleep is uncommouly profound, and these uneasy sensations great, the disease called the incubus or nightmare is produced. Here the desire of moving the body is painfully exerted; but the power of moving it, or volition, is incapable of action till we are awake."

In consequence of this misapprehension of the nature of the will, it is not easy to arrive at Darwin's ideas on the subject; and the attempt is rendered still more difficult from the fact that though he repeatedly states that volition is entirely suspended during sleep, he yet in the first part of the foregoing quotation makes an individual awake by the gradual exercise of the power of the will; and then in the last part of the same paragraph asserts that volition is incapable of action till sleep is over.

Mr. Dugald Stewart* contends that during sleep the power of volition is not suspended, but that those operations of the mind and body which depend on volition cease to be exercised. In his opinion the will loses its influence over all our powers both of mind and body in consequence of some physical alteration in the system which we

---

* Elements of the Philosophy of the Human Mind. Am. ed. Boston, 1818, vol. i. p. 184.

shall never probably be able to explain. To show in full the views of so distinguished a philosopher as Mr. Stewart, I quote the following extracts from his remarks on the subject:

"In order to illustrate this conclusion [the one above stated] a little further, it may be proper to remark that if the suspension of our voluntary operations in sleep be admitted as a fact, there are only two suppositions which can be formed regarding its cause. The one is that the power of volition is suspended; the other that the will loses its influence over those faculties of the mind and those members of the body which during our waking hours are subjected to its authority. If it can be shown then that the former supposition is not agreeable to fact, the truth of the latter seems to follow as a necessary consequence.

"1. That the power of volition is not suspended during sleep, appears from the efforts which we are conscious of making while in that situation. We dream, for instance, that we are in danger, and we attempt to call out for assistance. The attempt induced is in general unsuccessful, and the sounds that we emit are feeble and indistinct; but this only confirms, or rather is a necessary consequence of, the supposition that in sleep the connection between the will and our voluntary operations is disturbed or interrupted. The continuance of the power of volition is demonstrated by the effort, however ineffectual.

"In like manner, in the course of an alarming dream we are sometimes conscious of making an exertion to save ourselves by flight from an apprehended danger; but in spite of all our efforts we continue in bed. In such cases we commonly dream that we are attempting to escape and are prevented by some external obstacle; but the fact seems to be that the body is at that time not subject to the will. During the disturbed rest which we sometimes have when the body is indisposed, the mind appears to retain some power over it; but as even in these cases the motions which are made consist rather of a general agitation of the whole system than of the regular exertion of a particular member of it with a view to produce a certain effect, it is reasonable to conclude that in perfectly sound sleep the mind, although it retains the power of volition, retains no influence whatever over the bodily organs.

"In that particular condition of the system which is known by the name of *incubus*, we are conscious of a total want of power over the body; and I believe the common opinion is that it is this want of power which distinguishes the *incubus* from all the other modifications of sleep. But the more probable supposition seems to be that every species of sleep is accompanied with a suspension of the faculty of voluntary motion; and that the incubus has nothing peculiar in it but this—that the uneasy sensations which are produced by the accidental posture of the body, and which we find it impossible to remove by our own efforts, render us distinctly conscious of our incapacity to move. One thing is certain, that the instant of our awaking and of our recovering the command of our bodily organs is one and the same.

"2. The same conclusion is confirmed by a different view of the subject. It is probable, as was already observed, that when we are anxious to procure sleep the state into which we naturally bring the mind approaches to its state after sleep commences. Now it is manifest that the means which nature directs us to employ on such occasions is not to suspend the powers of volition, but to suspend the exertion of those powers whose exercise depends on volition. If it were necessary that volition should be suspended before we fall asleep, it would be impossible for us by our own efforts to hasten the moment of rest. The very supposition of such efforts is absurd, for it implies a continued will to suspend the acts of the will.

"According to the foregoing doctrine with respect to the state of the mind in sleep, the effort which is produced on our mental operations is strikingly analogous to that which is produced on our bodily powers. From the observations which have been already made, it is manifest that in sleep the body is in a very inconsiderable degree, if at all, subject to our command. The vital and involuntary motions, however, suffer no interruption, but go on as when we are awake, in consequence of the operation

9

of some cause unknown to us. In like manner it
would appear that those operations of the mind
which depend on our volition are suspended, while
certain other operations are at least occasionally
carried on. This analogy naturally suggests the
idea that all our mental operations which are independent of our will may continue during sleep; and
that the phenomena of dreaming may, perhaps, be
produced by these, diversified in their apparent ef-
feets in consequence of the suspension of our voluntary powers."

A very little reflection will suffice to convince
the reader that Mr. Stewart has altogether mistaken the nature of sleep. There is no evidence to
support his view that the body is not subject to the
action of the will during sleep. No change whatever is induced by this condition in the nerves or
muscles of the organism. The first are just as
capable as ever of conducting the nervous fluid, and
the muscles do not lose any of their contractile
power. The reason why voluntary movements are
not performed in sleep is simply because the will
does not act; and Mr. Stewart is again wrong in asserting that volition is not then suspended. We do
not will any actions when we are asleep. We imagine we do, and that is all. The difficulties which
encompass us in sleep are, it must be recollected,
purely imaginary, and the efforts we make to escape
from them are likewise the products of our fancy.
Herein lies the main error which Mr. Stewart has

committed. He appears to accept the dream for a reality, and to regard the seeming volitions which occur in it as actual facts; whereas they are all entirely fictitious.

An example will serve to make this point still clearer.

Not long since I dreamed that I stood upon a very high perpendicular table-land, at the foot of which flowed a river. I thought I experienced an irresistible desire to approach the brink and to look down. Had I been awake, such a wish would have been the very last to enter my mind, for I have an instinctive dread of standing on a height. I dreamed that I threw myself on my face and crawled to the edge of the cliff. I looked down at the stream, which scarcely appeared to be as wide as my hand, so great was the altitude upon which I was placed. As I looked I felt an overpowering impulse to crawl still farther and to throw myself into the water below. I imagined that I endeavored with all my will to resist this force, which appeared to be acting by means altogether external to my organism. My efforts, however, were all in vain. I could not control my movements, and gradually I was urged farther and farther over the brink, till at last I went down into the abyss below. As I struck the water I awoke with a start. During my imaginary struggle I thought I experienced all the emotions which such an event if real would have excited, and I was painfully conscious of my utter inability to escape

from the peril of my situation.   Here were circumstances such as, according to Mr. Stewart, demon
strate the activity of volition, but at the same time
show its inability to act upon the body.   But clearly
they show no such thing, for the imaginary volition
was to refrain from crawling over a precipice which
did not exist, and over which, therefore, I was not
hanging.   Such an act of the will if real, could not
in the very nature of the real conditions of the situation have been carried out—the volition was just
as imaginary as all the other circumstances of the
dream.

Again, it is not always the case that the imaginary
acts of the will are not executed during sleep; and
hence it would follow from Mr. Stewart's argument
that the power of the will over the body is not then
suspended.   Assuming for the moment that the
volitions of sleep are real, as Mr. Stewart supposes;
if it can be shown that they are satisfactorily performed, it results from his line of reasoning that
the will has power over the body during sleep.
Every one who has ever dreamed has at times had
his will carried out to his entire satisfaction.   He
has ridden horses when pursued, and has urged
them forward with whip and spur so as to escape
from his enemies.   Or he has executed the most
surprising feats both with his mind and body, and
has performed voluntary deeds which have excited
the admiration of all beholders.   Such acts are of
course entirely the product of the imagination, and

all the volitions which accompany them have no firmer basis than the unbridled fancy; but, according to Mr. Stewart, they would be evidence of the power of the will over the body,—a power which in reality does not exist; not, however, as Mr. Stewart supposes from any impediments in the nerves or muscles, but because it is never exerted.

So far as relates to movements performed during sleep, such as turning in bed and assuming more comfortable positions, they have nothing whatever to do with the will. They are dependent upon the action of the spinal cord, an organ that is never at rest, and the functions of which were not known as well when Dr. Darwin and Mr. Stewart wrote as they are now. The same is true of more complex and longer-continued actions, such as those already mentioned of individuals riding on horseback, or even walking, during sleep.

Cabanis* contends that the will is not entirely suspended during sleep; but, as will be perceived from the following quotation, he bases his argument upon the fact that movements are produced which he attributes erroneously to the action of the will, but which, like those previously referred to, are accomplished by the agency of the spinal cord. He says, speaking of the instances of persons walking while asleep:

"These rare cases are not the only ones in which

---

* Op. cit., t. ii. p. 376, et seq. Article Du Sommeil en particulier.

9*

during sleep movements are produced by what remains of the will; for it is by virtue of certain direct
sensations that a sleeping man moves his arm to
brush away the flies that may be on his face, that
he draws up the bedclothes so as to cover himself
carefully; or, as we have already remarked, that he
turns over and endeavors to find a more comfortable
position. It is the will which during sleep maintains the contraction of the sphincter of the bladder,
notwithstanding the effort of the urine to escape;
it is the same power which directs the action of the
arm in seeking for the *vase de nuit*, which knows
where to find it, and enables the individual to use it
for several minutes and to return it to its place without being awakened. Finally, it is not without reason that some physiologists have made the will
concur in the contraction of several muscles, the
movements of which are necessary to the maintenance of respiration during sleep."

All these movements, and many others of a similar character, are entirely spinal, and are altogether
independent of cerebral influence. Even when we
are awake, we constantly execute muscular actions
through the power of the spinal cord, when the
mind is intently occupied with other things. Take
for instance the example of a person playing on the
piano, and at the same time carrying on a conversation. Here the brain is engaged in the one act and
the spinal cord in the other. So long as the player
is not expert in the fingering of the instrument, he

cannot divert his attention from his performance; for the whole power of the mind is required for the proper appreciation and execution of the music. But after the spinal cord has become educated to the habit, and he has attained proficiency in the necessary manipulations, the mind is no longer required to control the actions and may be directed to other subjects. The arguments of Cabanis, therefore, in favor of the partial exercise of the will during sleep, are of no force.

But the power of the will over the muscles of the body is only one of the ways in which this faculty is shown. It regulates the thoughts and the manifestations of emotion when we are awake. How utterly incapable it is of any such action during sleep we all know. A gentleman, remarkable for the ability he possesses for controlling his feelings, tells me that when he is asleep he frequently weeps or laughs at imaginary events, which, if they really had occurred to him during wakefulness, would give rise to no such disturbance. He often desires to stop these emotional manifestations, but is entirely powerless to do so. Most individuals have had similar experiences.

The theory that the will is in action during sleep is, therefore, to my mind untenable. It has probably had its origin in the idea that confounds it with desire, from which it differs so markedly that it seems strange the distinction should ever fail of being made. Locke* points out very clearly the differences between the two faculties. In fact they may be exerted in directly opposite ways. Desire often precedes volition; but we all, at times, will acts which are contrary to our desire, and desire to perform others which we are unable to will.

Reid† writes with great perspicuity on this distinction between desire and will. He says:

"Desire and will agree in this, that both must have an object of which we must have some conception; and, therefore, both must be accompanied with some degree of understanding. But they differ in several things.

"The object of desire may be anything which appetite, passion, or affection leads us to pursue; it may be any event which we think good for us, or for those to whom we are well affected. I may desire meat or drink, or ease from pain. But to say that I will meat, or will drink, or will ease from pain, is not English. There is, therefore, a distinction in common language between desire and will. And the distinction is, that what we will must be an action and our own action; what we desire may not be our own action, it may be no action at all.

"A man desires that his children may be happy,

---

* An Essay Concerning Human Understanding, chapter xxi. section 30.

† Essays on the Powers of the Human Mind, vol. iii. Edinburgh, 1803, p. 77.

and that they may behave well. Their being happy is no action at all; their behaving well is not his action but theirs.

"With regard to our own actions, we may desire what we do not will, and will what we do not desire; nay, what we have a great aversion to.

"A man athirst has a strong desire to drink; but for some particular reason he determines not to gratify his desire. A judge from a regard to justice and to the duty of his office dooms a criminal to die; while, from humanity or particular affection, he desires that he should live. A man for health may take a nauseous draught, for which he has no desire, but a great aversion. Desire, therefore, even when its object is some action of our own, is only an incitement to will; but it is not volition. The determination of the mind may be not to do what we desire to do. But as desire is often accompanied by will, we are apt to overlook the distinction between them."

That desire is manifested during sleep there can be no doubt; and Mr. Stewart, although insisting as he does on the distinction between this faculty and volition, confounds them in his remarks already quoted. A person suffering from nightmare has a most intense desire to escape from his imaginary troubles. In my own dream, to which reference has been made, my desire to restrain myself from crawling over the precipice was exerted to the utmost; but the will could not be brought into action. Darwin,* when he says that in nightmare "the *desire* of moving the body is painfully exerted, but the *power of moving it, or volition*, is incapable of action till we awake," makes the proper distinction between desire and will; but, as I have already shown, confounds the latter with another very different faculty.

From the foregoing observations it will be seen that during sleep the three great divisions of the mind are differently affected.

1. Feeling, embracing sensation and emotion, is suspended, so far as the first is concerned; but is in full action as regards the second. We do not see, hear, smell, taste or enjoy the sense of touch in sleep, although the brain may be aroused into activity and we may awake through the excitations conveyed to it by the special senses. The emotions have full play, unrestrained by the will and governed only by the imagination.

2. The Will or Volition is entirely suspended.

3. The Thought or Intellect is variously affected in its different powers. The imagination is active, and the memory may be exercised to a great extent; but the judgment, perception, conception, abstraction, and reason are weakened, and sometimes altogether lost.

---

* Op. cit., p. 155.

CHAPTER V.

THE PHYSIOLOGY OF DREAMS.

THE subject of the foregoing chapter is so intimately connected with the phenomena of dreaming, and I have expressed my views in regard to it at such length, that but few psychological points remain to be considered in the present discussion. What I have to say, therefore, in regard to the physiology of dreaming must be read in connection with the chapter on *"The State of the Mind during Sleep,"* in order that the whole matter may be fully understood.

It is contended by some writers that the mind is never at rest, and that even during the most profound sleep dreams take place, which are either forgotten immediately, or which make no impression on the memory. That this view is erroneous is, I think, very evident. If it were correct, the first object of sleep—rest for the brain—would not be attained. We all know how fatigued we are, and how indisposed to exertion the brain is, after a night of continued dreaming, and we can easily imagine what would be the consequences if such a condition were kept up night after night. To say that we really do dream not only every night, but every instant of the night, in fact always and continually when we sleep, but that we forget our dreams as soon as they are formed, remembering solely those which are most vivid, is making assertions which not only are without proof, but which are impossible of proof. For if, as Locke* remarks, the sleeping man on awaking has no recollection of his thoughts, it is very certain that no one else can recollect them for him.

The observations of Locke on this point are extremely appropriate, and, to my mind, very philosophical and logical. After insisting that, sleeping or waking, a man cannot think without being sensible of it, he says :†

"I grant that the soul of a waking man is never without thought, because it is the condition of being awake; but whether sleeping without dreaming be not an affection of the whole man, mind as well as body, may be worth a waking man's consideration, it being hard to conceive that anything should think and not be conscious of it. If the soul doth think in a sleeping man without being conscious of it, I ask, whether during such thinking it has any pleasure or pain, or be capable of happiness or misery? I am sure the man is not, any more than the bed or earth he lies on, for to be happy or miserable without

---

* An Essay Concerning the Human Understanding, book ii. section 17.

† Op. et loc. cit., section 11.

being conscious of it seems to me utterly inconsistent and impossible. Or if it be possible that the soul can, while the body is sleeping, have its thinkings, enjoyments, and concerns, its pleasure or pain, about which the man is not conscious of nor partakes in, it is certain that Socrates asleep and Socrates awake is not the same person; but his soul when he sleeps and Socrates the man, consisting of body and soul when he is waking, are two persons, since waking Socrates has no knowledge of or concernment for that happiness or misery of his soul which it enjoys alone by itself while he sleeps without perceiving anything of it, any more than he has for the happiness or misery of a man in the Indies whom he knows not; for if we take wholly away all consciousness of our actions and sensations, especially of pleasure and pain, and the concernment that accompanies it, it will be hard to know wherein to place personal identity.''

In a subsequent section of the same chapter, Locke asserts that most men pass a great part of their lives without dreaming, and that he once knew a scholar who had no bad memory, who told him he had never dreamed in his life till after the occurrence of a fever in the twenty-fifth or twenty-sixth year of his age.

Examples of persons who have not ordinarily dreamed are adduced by the ancient writers. Pliny*

---

* Historia Naturalis, lib. x. cap. lxxv., "De Somno Animalium."

refers to men who never dreamed. Plutarch* alludes to the case of Cleon, who, in living to an advanced age, had yet never dreamed; and Suetonius† declares that before the murder of his mother he had never dreamed.

A lady who was under my care for a serious nervous affection declared to me that she never had had but one dream in her life, and that was after receiving a severe fall in which she struck her head.

And yet, notwithstanding the experience of every one that sleep often happens without the accompaniment of dreams, the great majority of writers hold the view that the brain is never at rest. Doubtless this opinion has its origin partly in the doctrine that the mind is a something altogether independent of and superior to the brain. They appear to be incapable of appreciating the fact that when the brain is in a state of complete repose there can be no mental manifestation, and that all intellectual phenomena are the results of cerebral activity. Another cause for their belief is the fact that they make no distinction between dreaming and thinking, whereas it is very evident that the two are not to be placed in the same category. Thinking is an *action* which requires cerebral effort, and which is undertaken with a determinate purpose. We will to think, and we think what we please; but it is very different with

---

* De defectu oraculorum.
† De Vita, xii. Cæsarum, Nero, cap. xlvi.

our dreams, which come and go without any power on our part to regulate or direct them. To think requires all the faculties of the mind; to dream necessitates only the memory and the imagination. In thinking, the brain is active in all its parts; in dreaming, it is nearly entirely quiescent.

Writers who contend for the doctrine of constant mental activity regard the brain as the organ or tool of the mind, a structure which the mind makes use of in order to manifest itself. Such a theory is certain to lead them into difficulties, and is contrary to all the teaching of physiology. The full discussion of this question would be out of place here; I will, therefore, only state that this work is written from the stand-point of regarding the mind as nothing more than the result of cerebral action. Just as a good liver secretes good bile, a good candle gives good light, and good coal a good fire, so does a good brain give a good mind. When the brain is quiescent there is no mind.

Lemoine* begins his chapter "*On the State of the Mind during Sleep*" with the assertion that "there is no sleep for the mind." He is obliged, however, to admit that "when the organs of the body are benumbed by sleep, the mind appears to be in a particular state; it seems to be submitted to other laws than those which govern it during wakefulness; it

---

* Op. cit., p. 63.

seems to have lost for a time its most precious faculties."

During sleep the mind is, as he supposes, in a particular state, for, as has been shown in the previous
chapter, it has lost many of its chief parts. The
laws which govern it are, however, the same which
always regulate it. The body upon which their
power is primarily exercised—the brain—is not in
the same condition during sleep as during wakefulness, and hence the differences in the evidences of
cerebral activity.

Sir William Hamilton* is generally considered to
have determined affirmatively the question of the
continuance of the action of the brain during sleep.
He caused himself to be aroused from sleep at intervals through the night, and invariably found that he
was disturbed from a dream, the particulars of which
he could always distinctly recollect. But a full
knowledge of the subject he was investigating
would have sufficed to convince Sir William that
the conclusion he drew from his experiments was
altogether fallacious. It is well known that dreams
are excited by strong impressions made upon the
senses, or by irritations arising in the internal
organs. Thus Baron Trenck relates that when confined in his dungeon he suffered the pangs of hunger
almost continually, and that his dreams at night
were always of delicate meats and sumptuous re-

* Lectures on Metaphysics, vol. i. p. 323.

pasts, spread before him on luxuriously-furnished tables. The mere excitation of waking a sleeping person is generally sufficient to give rise to a dream. Maury, in his very interesting work, to which reference has already been made, and which will hereafter be more specifically considered, adduces many examples of dreams produced by sensorial impressions. I have myself performed many experiments with reference to this point, and have generally found ample confirmation of Maury's investigations. It may therefore, I think, be assumed, without any violence to the actual facts of the cases, that the brain is not always in action, and that there are times when we sleep without dreaming.

In the previous chapter the idea is sought to be conveyed that we originate nothing in our dreams. We may conceive of things which never existed, or of which we have heard or read, but the images we make of them are either composed of elements familiar to us, or else are based upon ideal representations which we have formed in our waking moments. Thus, before the discovery of America no Europeans ever dreamed of American Indians, for the reason that nothing existed within their knowledge which could give any idea of the appearance of such human beings. It is possible that Columbus and his companions may have dreamed of the continent of which they were in search and of its natives, but the images formed of the latter must necessarily have resembled other beings they had seen, or which

10*

they had heard described. After the discovery, how-ever, it was no unusual thing for the Spaniards and others to have correct images of Indians appear to them in their dreams.

Dreams, therefore, must have a foundation, and this is either impressions made upon the mind at some previous period, or produced during sleep by bodily sensations. These impressions, however they may be formed, are subjected to the unrestrained influence of the imagination.

At first sight it may seem that we often have dreams not excited by actual sensations, and which have no relation to any events of our lives, or any ideas which have passed through our minds, but thorough investigation will invariably reveal the existence of an association between the dream and some such ideas or events. For instance, a few nights ago I dreamed that a gentleman, a friend of mine, had invented what he called a "dog-cart am-bulance," a vehicle which he declared was the best ever made for the transportation of sick or wounded men. On awaking, all the particulars were fresh in my mind, but I could not for some time perceive why I had had such a dream. At last I recollected that the morning before a gentleman had given me a very full description of Prospect Park, in Brook-lyn. The friend of whom I dreamed has charge of the construction of this Park. His presence was, therefore, fully explained, and as dog-carts are driven in parks, this link was also accounted for. The ambulance part was due to the fact that I had that same morning found the card of a gentleman upon my table who really had invented an ambulance. The imagination had, therefore, taken these data supplied by the memory, and had combined them into the incongruous web constituting my dream.

Dreams are also frequently built upon circumstances which have transpired many years previously, and which have long since apparently passed from our recollection. A very striking instance of this kind is related by Abercrombie,* on the authority of Sir Walter Scott.

" Mr. R. J. Rowland, a gentleman of landed property in the vale of Gala, was prosecuted for a very considerable sum, the accumulated arrears of teind (tithe), for which he was said to be indebted to a noble family the titulars (lay impropriators of the tithe). Mr. R. was strongly impressed with the belief that his father had, by a form of process peculiar to the law of Scotland, purchased these teinds from the titular, and, therefore, that the present prosecution was groundless. But after an industrious search among his father's papers, an investigation of the public records, and a careful inquiry among all persons who had transacted law business for his father, no evidence could be discovered to support his defense. The period was now near at hand when he conceived

---

* Inquiries Concerning the Intellectual Powers and the Investigation of Truth. Tenth edition. London, 1840, p. 283.

the loss of his lawsuit to be inevitable, and he had formed his determination to ride to Edinburgh next day, and make the best bargain he could in the way of compromise.   He went to bed with this resolution, and, with all the circumstances of the case floating upon his mind, had a dream to the following purpose.   His father, who had been many years dead, appeared to him, he thought, and asked him why he was disturbed in his mind.   In dreams men are not surprised at such apparitions.   Mr. R. thought that he informed his father of the cause of his distress, adding that the payment of a considerable sum of money was the more unpleasant to him, because he had a stray consciousness that it was not due, though he was unable to recover any evidence in support of his belief.   'You are right, my son,' replied the paternal shade; 'I did acquire right to these teinds, for payment of which you are now prosecuted.   The papers relating to the transaction are in the hands of Mr. ——, a writer (or attorney), who is now retired from professional business, and resides at Inveresk, near Edinburgh.   He was a person whom I employed on that occasion for a particular reason, but who never, on any other occasion, transacted business on my account.   It is very possible,' pursued the vision, 'that Mr. —— may have forgotten a matter which is now of a very old date; but you may call it to his recollection by this token— that when I came to pay his account there was difficulty in getting change for a Portugal piece of gold, and that we were forced to drink out the balance at a tavern.'

"Mr. R. awaked in the morning with all the events of the vision impressed on his mind, and thought it worth while to ride across the country to Inveresk, instead of going straight to Edinburgh. When he came there he waited on the gentleman mentioned in the dream, a very old man; without saying anything of the vision, he inquired whether he remembered having conducted such a matter for his deceased father. The old gentleman could not at first bring the circumstance to his recollection, but, on mention of the Portugal piece of gold, the whole returned upon his memory; he made an immediate search for the papers and recovered them, so that Mr. R. carried to Edinburgh the documents necessary to gain the cause which he was on the verge of losing."

A friend has related to me some circumstances in his own case similar to the above, and illustrating the same points. In the course of his practice as a lawyer, it became necessary for him to ascertain the exact age of a client, who was also his cousin. Their grandfather had been a rather eccentric personage, who had taken a great deal of notice of both his grandsons—his only direct descendants. He died when they were boys. My friend often told his cousin that if his grandfather were alive there would be no difficulty at getting at the desired information, and that he had a dim recollection of having seen a record kept by the old gentleman, and of there being some peculiarity about it which he could not recall. Several months elapsed, and he had given up the idea of attempting to discover the facts of which he had been in search, when, one night, he dreamed that his grandfather came to him and said: "You have been trying to find out when J—— was born; don't you recollect that one afternoon when we were fishing I read you some lines from an Elzevir Horace, and showed you how I had made a family record out of the work by inserting a number of blank leaves at the end? Now, as you know, I devised my library to the Rev. —— ——. I was a d——d fool for giving him books which he will never read! Get the Horace, and you will discover the exact hour at which J—— was born." In the morning all the particulars of this dream were fresh in my friend's memory. The reverend gentleman lived in a neighboring city; my friend took the first train, found the copy of Horace, and at the end the pages constituting the family record, exactly as had been described to him in the dream. By no effort of his memory, however, could he recollect the incidents of the fishing excursion.

Dr. Macnish,* in stating his opinion that dreams are uniformly the resuscitation or re-embodiment of thoughts which have formerly, in some shape or

---

* Op. cit., p. 10.

other, occupied the mind, relates the following example from his own experience:

"I lately dreamed that I walked upon the banks of the great canal in the neighborhood of Glasgow. On the side opposite to that on which I was, and within a few feet of the water, stood the splendid portico of the Royal Exchange. A gentleman whom I knew was standing upon one of the steps, and we spoke to each other. I then lifted a large stone and poised it in my hand, when he said that he was certain I could not throw it to a certain spot, which he pointed out. I made the attempt, and fell short of the mark. At this moment a well-known friend came up, whom I knew to excel at *putting* the stone; but, strange to say, he had lost both his legs, and walked upon wooden substitutes. This struck me as exceedingly curious, for my impression was that he had only lost one leg, and had but a single wooden one. At my desire he took up the stone, and, without difficulty, threw it beyond the point indicated by the gentleman upon the opposite side of the canal. The absurdity of this dream is extremely glaring, and yet, on strictly analyzing it, I find it to be wholly composed of ideas which passed through my mind on the previous day, assuming a new and ridiculous arrangement. I can compare it to nothing but to cross reading in the newspapers, or to that well-known amusement which consists in putting a number of sentences, each written on a separate piece of paper, into a hat, shaking the whole, then taking

them out, one by one, as they come, and seeing
what kind of medley the heterogeneous compound
will make when thus fortuitously put together. For
instance, I had, on the above day, taken a walk to
the canal along with a friend. On returning from
it, I pointed out to him a spot where a new road was
forming, and where, a few days before, one of the
workmen had been overwhelmed by a quantity of
rubbish falling upon him, which fairly chopped off
one of his legs, and so much damaged the other
that it was feared amputation would be necessary.
Near this very spot there is a park, in which, about
a month previously, I practiced throwing the stone.
On passing the Exchange, on my way home, I expressed regret at the lowness of its situation, and
remarked what a fine effect the portico would have
were it placed upon more elevated ground. Such
were the previous circumstances, and let us see how
they bear upon the dream. In the first place, the
canal appeared before me. 2. Its situation is an
elevated one. 3. The portico of the Exchange occurring to my mind as being placed too low became
associated with the elevation of the canal, and I
placed it close by on a similar altitude. 4. The
gentleman I had been walking with was the same
whom in the dream I saw standing upon the steps
of the portico. 5. Having related to him the story
of the man who lost one limb and had a chance of
losing another, this idea brings before me a friend
with a pair of wooden legs, who, moreover, appears

in connection with putting the stone, as I knew him to excel at that exercise. There is only one other element in the dream which the preceding events will not account for, and that is the surprise at the individual referred to having more than one wooden leg. But why should he have even one, seeing that in reality he is limbed like other people? This also I can account for. Two years ago he slightly injured his knee while leaping a ditch, and I remember jocularly advising him to get it cut off. I am particular in illustrating this point with regard to dreams, for I hold that if it were possible to analyze them all, they would invariably be found to stand in the same relation to the waking state as the above specimen. The more diversified and incongruous the character of a dream, and the more remote from the period of its occurrence the circumstances which suggested it, the more difficult does its analysis become; and, in point of fact, this process may be impossible, so totally are the elements of the dream often dissevered from their original sense, and so ludicrously huddled together."

A dream which Professor Maas,* of Halle, relates as having occurred to himself, affords an excellent example of the dependence of dreams upon actual events, and shows how these latter are distorted and perverted by the imagination of the sleeper.

* Quoted in Dendy's Philosophy of Mystery. London, 1841, p. 225.

"I dreamed once," he says, "that the Pope visited me. He commanded me to open my desk, and he carefully examined all the papers it contained. While he was thus employed, a very sparkling diamond fell out of his triple crown into my desk, of which, however, neither of us took any notice. As soon as the Pope had withdrawn I retired to bed, but was soon obliged to rise on account of a thick smoke, the cause of which I had yet to learn. Upon examination I discovered that the diamond had set fire to the papers in my desk, and burned them to ashes."

In analyzing the circumstances which gave rise to this dream, Professor Maas relates the following events, which constituted its basis:

"On the preceding evening I was visited by a friend with whom I had a lively conversation upon Joseph II.'s suppression of monasteries and convents. With this idea, though I did not become conscious of it in the dream, was associated the visit which the Pope publicly paid the Emperor Joseph, at Vienna, in consequence of the measures taken against the clergy; and with this again was combined, however faintly, the representation of the visit which had been paid me by my friend. These two events were, by the subreasoning faculty, compounded into one, according to the established rule —that things which agree in their parts also correspond as to the whole; hence the Pope's visit was changed into a visit paid to me. The subreasoning faculty, then, in order to account for this extraordinary visit, fixed upon that which was the most important object in my room—namely, the desk, or rather the papers which it contained. That a diamond fell out of the triple crown was a collateral association, which was owing merely to the representation of the desk. Some days before, when opening the desk, I had broken the crystal of my watch, which I held in my hand, and the fragments fell among the papers; hence no further attention was paid to the diamond being a representation of a collateral series of things. But afterwards the representation of the sparkling stone was again excited, and became the prevailing idea; hence it determined the succeeding association. On account of its similarity it excited the representation of fire, with which it was confounded; hence arose fire and smoke. But in the event the writings only were burned, not the desk itself, to which, being of comparatively little value, the attention was not directed."

Feuchtersleben* takes the same view of dreaming as that enunciated in this chapter. Thus he says:

Dreaming is nothing more than the occupation of the mind in sleep with the pictorial world of fancy. As the closed or quiescent senses afford it no materials, the mind, ever active, must make use of the store which memory retains; but as its motor influence is likewise organically impeded, it cannot

---

* The Principles of Medical Psychology, etc. Sydenham Society Translation. London, 1847, p. 163.

independently dispose of this store. Thus arises a condition in which the mind looks, as it were, on the play of the images within itself, and manifests only a faint or partial reaction."

Locke[*] contends that "the dreams of a sleeping man are all made up of the waking man's ideas oddly put together."

Observation and reflection show us that the mind originates nothing during sleep; it merely remembers—and often in the most chaotic manner—the thoughts, the fancies, the impressions which have been imagined or received by the individual when awake. Sometimes ideas are reproduced in dreams exactly as they have occurred to us in our waking moments, and this may take place night after night with scarcely the alteration of a single circumstance. A friend informs me that he is very subject to dreams of this character, and that on some occasions the repetition has taken place as many as a dozen times.

A very striking instance of this kind occurred to me a few years since, and made a deep impression on my mind. I had just read Schiller's ode to Laura, as translated by Sir E. Bulwer Lytton, beginning,

" Who and what gave to me the wish to woo thee ?"

and admired it as a striking piece of versification conveying some noted philosophical ideas in a forci-

* Op. cit., book ii. sec. 17.

ble and beautiful manner. The following night I had a very vivid dream of a condition of pre-existence, in which I imagined myself to be. The connection between the dream and the poem I had been reading was sufficiently well marked, and did not astonish me. I was, however, surprised to find that the next night I had exactly the same dream, and that it was repeated three times subsequently on consecutive nights.

The dependence of dreams upon ideas which we have had when awake was well known to the ancients. Thus Lucius Accius,* a poet who lived more than a hundred and fifty years before the Christian era, says :

" Quae in vita usurpant homines, cogitant, curant, vident
Quaeque agunt vigilantes, agitantque casi cui in somno accidant,
*　　*　　*　　*　　*　　*　　Minus mirum est."

Lucretius† declares that during sleep we are amused with things which have made us weep when awake; that circumstances which have pleased us are recalled to our minds; that objects are presented to us which occupied our thoughts long before; and that recent events appear still more vividly before us.

Petronius Arbiter‡ cites Epicurus to the same

---

* Cited by M. l'Abbé Richard in *La Théorie des Songes*. Paris, 1766, p. 32.

† De Rerum Natura, l. iv. v. 959.

‡ Satyricon. Bohu's edition. London, 1854, p. 307.

11*

effect. Tryphæna having declared that she had had a dream in which there appeared to her the image of Neptune she had seen at Baiæ, "Hence you may perceive," observed Eumolpus, "what a divine man is Epicurus, who so ingeniously ridiculed these sports of fancy.

"When in a dream presented to our view
Those airy forms appear so like the true,
No prescient shrine, no god the vision sends,
But every breast its own delusion lends.
For when soft sleep the body wraps in ease,
And from the inactive mass the fancy frees,
What most by day affects, at night returns;
Thus he who shakes proud states, and cities burns,
Sees showers of darts, forced lines, disordered wings,
Blood-reeking fields, and deaths of vanquished kings;
He that by day litigious knots untied,
And charmed the drowsy bench to either side,
By night a crowd of cringing clients sees,
Smiles on the fools and kindly takes their fees;
The miser hides his wealth, new treasure finds;
Through echoing woods his horn the huntsman winds;
The sailor's dream wild scenes of wreck describes;
The wanton lays her snares; the adultress bribes;
Hounds in full cry, in sleep, the hare pursue;
And hapless wretches their old griefs renew."*

It is related of an ancient tyrant that one of his courtiers described to him a dream in which the

---

* In the above quotation I have slightly altered Kelly's version in Bohn's edition of Petronius. The original Latin is fully as forcible and true to nature as the translation.

courtier had assassinated his master. "You could not," exclaimed the tyrant, "have dreamed this without having previously thought of it," and then ordered his immediate execution.

Now besides this foundation of dreams upon circumstances which have transpired during our waking moments, they may arise, as has already been intimated, from impressions made upon the mind during sleep. Sensations may be so intense as to be partially appreciated by the brain, and yet not strong enough to cause sleep to be interrupted. In such cases the imagination seizes the imperfect perception and weaves it into a tissue of incongruous fancies, which, however, generally bear a more or less definite relation to the character of the sensorial impression. Many examples of dreams thus produced are on record, and many others have come under my own observation. The interest which attaches to phenomena of this character must be my excuse for quoting some of the more remarkable instances of this kind which have been brought to my attention.

The following are related by Abercrombie :*

During the alarm excited in Edinburgh by the apprehension of a French invasion almost every man was a soldier, and all things had been arranged in expectation of the landing of the enemy. The first notice was to be given by the firing of a gun from

---

* Op. cit., p. 275, et seq.

the Castle, and this was to be followed by a chain of signals calculated to arouse the country. The gentleman to whom the dream occurred was a zealous volunteer, and, being in bed between two and three o'clock in the morning, dreamt of hearing the signal gun. He imagined that he went at once to the Castle, witnessed the proceeding for displaying the signals, and saw and heard all the preparations for the assemblage of the troops. At this time he was roused by his wife, who awoke in a fright, in consequence of a similar dream. The origin of both dreams was ascertained in the morning to be the noise produced by the falling of a pair of tongs in the room above.

A gentleman dreamt that he had enlisted as a soldier, joined his regiment, deserted, was apprehended, carried back, condemned to be shot, and at last led out to execution. At this instant a gun was fired, and he awoke, to find that a noise in the adjoining room had both produced the dream and awakened him.

The next is a very extraordinary case.

The subject was an officer in the expedition to Louisburg, in 1758. During his passage in the transport his companions were in the habit of amusing themselves at his expense. They could produce in him any kind of dream by whispering in his ear, especially if this was done by a friend with whose voice he was familiar. Once they conducted him through the whole process of a quarrel which ended in a duel, and when the parties were supposed to have met a pistol was put into his hand, which he fired, and was awakened by the report. On another occasion they found him asleep on the top of a locker in the cabin, when they made him believe he had fallen overboard, and exhorted him to save himself by swimming. Then they told him that a shark was pursuing him, and entreated him to dive for his life. He instantly did so, and with so much force as to throw himself from the locker upon the cabin floor, by which he was much bruised, and awakened of course. After the landing of the army at Louisburg, his friends found him one day asleep in his tent, and evidently much annoyed by the cannonading. They then made him believe that he was engaged, when he exhibited great fear, and showed a decided disposition to run away. Against this they remonstrated, but at the same time increased his fears by imitating the groans of the wounded and the dying; and when he asked, as he often did, who was hit, they named his particular friends. At last they told him that the man next himself in his company had fallen, when he instantly sprang from his bed, rushed out of his tent, and was roused from his danger and his dream by falling over the tent-cords.

A friend informs me that he has a brother who will carry on a conversation with any person who whispers to him in his sleep, and that his emotions are then very readily excited by any pitiful story that may be told him.   Upon awaking, he has a distinct recollection of his dreams, which are always connected with the ideas communicated.

I recollect very distinctly the particulars of a dream which I had several years since, and which was due to an impression conveyed to the brain through the ear   The dream also illustrates the point previously brought forward, that a definite conception of time does not enter into the phenomena of dreams.

I dreamed that I had taken passage in a steamboat from St. Louis to New Orleans.   Among the passengers was a man who had all the appearance of being very ill with consumption.   He looked more like a ghost than a human being, and moved noiselessly among the passengers, noticing no one, though attracting the attention of all.   For several days nothing was said between him and any one, till one morning, as we approached Baton Rouge, he came to where I was sitting on the guards and began a conversation by asking me what time it was.   I took out my watch, when be instantly took it from my hand and opened it.   "I, too, once had a watch " he said; "but see what I am now."   With these words he threw aside the large cloak he habitually wore, and I saw that his ribs were entirely bare of skin and flesh.   He then took my watch, and, inserting it between his ribs, said it would make a very good heart.   Continuing his conversation he told me that he had resolved to blow up the vessel

the next day, but that as I had been the means of
supplying him with a heart he would save my life.
"When you hear the whistle blow," he said, "jump
overboard, for in an instant afterward the boat will
be in atoms." I thanked him, and he left me. All
that day and the next I endeavored to acquaint my
fellow-passengers with the fate in store for them, but
discovered that I had lost the faculty of speech. I tried
to write, but found that my hands were paralyzed.
In fact I could adopt no means to warn them. While
I was making these ineffectual efforts, I heard the
whistle of the engine; I rushed to the side of the
boat to plunge overboard, and awoke. The whistle
of a steam saw-mill near my house had just begun to
sound, and had awakened me. My whole dream
had been excited by it, and could not have occupied
more than a few seconds.

The following account* shows how a dream may
be set in action by the sense of smell.

"On one occasion during my residence at Bir-
mingham I had to attend many patients at Coventry,
and for their accommodation I visited that place
one day in every week. My temporary residence
was at a druggist's shop in the market-place. Having
on one occasion, now to be mentioned, a more than
usual number of engagements, I was obliged to remain one night, and a bed was provided for me at
the residence of a cheesemonger in the same locality.

* Journal of Psychological Medicine. July, 1856.

The house was very old, the rooms very low, and the street very narrow. It was summer-time, and during the day the cheesemaker had unpacked a box or barrel of strong old American cheese; the very street was impregnated with the odor. At night, jaded with my professional labors, I went to my dormitory, which seemed filled with a strong, cheesy atmosphere, which affected my stomach greatly, and quite disturbed the biliary secretions. I tried to produce a more agreeable atmosphere to my olfactory sense by smoking cigars, but did not succeed. At length, worn out with fatigue, I tried to sleep, and should have succeeded, but for a time another source of annoyance prevented me doing so; for in an old wall behind my head, against which my ancient bed stood, there were numerous rats gnawing away in real earnest. The crunching they made was indeed terrific, and I resisted the drowsy god from a dread that these voracious animals would make a forcible entrance, and might take personal liberties with my flesh.

"But at length 'tired nature' ultimately so overpowered me that I slept in a sort of fever. I was still breathing the cheesy atmosphere, and this, associated with the marauding rats, so powerfully affected my imagination that a most horrid dream was the consequence. I fancied myself in some barbarous country, where, being charged with a political offense, I was doomed to be incarcerated in a large cheese. And although this curious prison-house seemed most oppressive, it formed but part of my sufferings; for scarcely had I become reconciled to my probable fate than to my horror an army of rats attacked the monster cheese, and soon they seemed to have effected an entrance, and began to fix themselves in numbers upon my naked body. The agony I endured was increased by the seeming impossibility to drive them away, and, fortunately for my sanity, I awoke, but with a hot head and throbbing temples, and a sense of nausea from the extremely strong odor of the cheese."

I have on two occasions that I recollect had dreams which were due to odors. On one of them the smell of gas escaping in the room excited the dream of a chemical laboratory; on the other the smell of burning cloth caused me to dream of a laundry, and of one of the women ironing a blanket, which she scorched with a hot iron. A lady informs me that a similar odor produced in her a dream of the house being on fire and the impossibility of her escaping by reason of all her clothes being burned up.

Dreams are very readily excited through impressions made on the special nerves of sensation. Instances are given of persons sleeping with bottles of hot water applied to their feet dreaming of walking on burning lava, or some other hot substance. A patient related to me the particulars of a dream which occurred to him while he was asleep with a vessel of hot water applied to the soles of his feet.

12

He had, just before going to sleep, read in the evening paper an account of the capture of an English gentleman by Italian brigands.   He dreamt that while crossing the Rocky Mountains he had been attacked by two Mexicans, who, after a long fight, had succeeded in taking him alive.   They conveyed him very hurriedly to their camp, which was situated in a deep gorge.   Here they told him that unless he revealed to them the means of making gold from copper they would submit him to torture.   In vain he plead ignorance of any such process.   Pulling off his boots and stockings they held his naked feet to the fire till he shrieked with agony, and awoke to find that the blanket which was wrapped around the tin vessel containing the hot water had become disarranged, and that his feet were in direct contact with the hot metal.

In another case, that of a lady whose lower limbs were paralyzed, artificial heat was applied during the night to her feet.   Frequently her dreams had reference to this circumstance.   On one occasion she dreamed that she was transformed into a bear, and was being taught to dance by being made to stand on hot plates of iron.   On another, that the house was on fire, and that the floors were so hot as to burn her feet in her efforts to escape.   Again, that she was wading through a stream of water which came from a hot spring in the Central Park.

Another patient, a lady, subject to neuralgic attacks of great severity, frequently had the lancinating pains give rise to dreams in which she was stabbed with daggers, cut with knives, torn with pincers, etc.

Not long since I had an attack of erysipelas, in which the disease included the head and face. The pain was not severe, and yet it was sufficient to give rise to the following dream :

I dreamed that I was taking a cold bath, and that while thus engaged a Turk, armed with a pair of long pincers, came into the room and began to pull the hair out of my head. I remonstrated, but was unable to offer any material resistance, for the reason that the water in which I was lying suddenly froze, leaving me imbedded in a solid cake of ice. In order to facilitate his operations, the Turk sponged my head with boiling water, and then, finding the use of the pincers rather slow work, shaved the hair off with a red-hot razor. He then rubbed an ointment on the naked scalp, composed of sulphur, phosphorus, and turpentine, to which he immediately applied fire. Taking me in his arms he rushed down stairs into the street, lighting his way with the flame from my burning head. He had not gone far before he fell down in a fit, and in his struggles gave me a severe blow between the eyes which instantly deprived me of sight.

When I awoke in the morning I had a very distinct recollection of this dream. The incidents were in part due to the fact that I had, two or three days previously, been reading an account of the insanity of Mohammed, and of his being subject to attacks of epilepsy.

The sense of taste is not, for obvious reasons, so productive of dreams as the other senses, but the experiments of M. Maury and myself, to which fuller reference will presently be made, show that strong excitations made upon it are transmitted to the brain; and the following instance, which has recently come under my immediate observation, is an interesting case in point.

A young lady had, in her early childhood, contracted the habit of going to sleep with her thumb in her mouth. She had tried for several years to break herself of the practice, but all her attempts were in vain, for even when by strong mental effort she succeeded in getting to sleep without the usual accompaniment, it was not long before the unruly member was in its accustomed place. Finally she hit upon the plan of covering the offending thumb with extract of aloes just before she went to bed, hoping that if she put it into her mouth she would instantly awake. But she slept on through the night, and in the morning found her thumb in her mouth and all the extract of aloes sucked off. During the night, however, she dreamed that she was crossing the ocean in a steamer made of wormwood, and that the vessel was furnished throughout with the same material. The plates, the dishes, tumblers, chairs, tables, etc. were all of wormwood, and the emanations so pervaded all parts of the ship that it was impossible to breathe without tasting the bitterness. Everything that she ate or drank was likewise, from being in contact with wormwood, so impregnated with the flavor that the taste was overpowering. When she arrived at Havre she asked for a glass of water for the purpose of washing the taste from her mouth, but they brought her an infusion of wormwood, which she gulped down because she was thirsty, though the sight of it excited nausea. She went to Paris and consulted a famous physician, M. Sauve Moi, begging him to do something which would extract the wormwood from her body. He told her there was but one remedy, and that was ox gall. This he gave her by the pound, and in a few weeks the wormwood was all gone, but the ox gall had taken its place, and was fully as bitter and disagreeable. To get rid of the ox gall she was advised to take counsel of the Pope. She accordingly went to Rome, and obtained an audience of the Holy Father. He told her that she must make a pilgrimage to the plain where the pillar of salt stood, into which Lot's wife was transformed, and must eat a piece of the salt as big as her thumb. During her journey in search of the pillar of salt she endured a great many sufferings, but finally triumphed over all obstacles, and reached the object of her journey. What part to take was now the question. After a good deal of deliberation she reasoned that as she had a bad habit of sucking her thumb, it would be very philosophical to break off this part from the statue, and thus not only get cured of the bitterness in her mouth, but also of her failing. She did so, put the piece of salt into her mouth, and awoke to find that she was sucking her own thumb.

It might be supposed that the brain during sleep is not excitable through the sense of sight. Many examples, however, are on record of dreams being thus produced, and several very interesting cases have come under my own observation. Among them are the following:

A gentleman of a nervous and irritable disposition informed me that he had dreamed of being in heaven and being dazzled by the brilliancy of everything around him. So great was the light that he hastened to escape from the pain which it caused in his eyes. In the efforts which he made he struck his head against the bedpost, and awoke to find that the fire which he had left smouldering on the hearth had kindled into a bright flame, the light from which fell full in his face.

Another, who had been under my care for epilepsy, dreamed that his room was entered by burglars, and that with lighted candles in their hands they were searching his drawers and trunks. He related his dream the following morning, and was told by his mother that she had gone into his room the previous night, and had held a lighted candle close to his face in order to see whether or not he was sound asleep.

No one has more philosophically studied the mode

of production of dreams than M. Maury* in his remarkable work to which reference has already been
made. I propose, therefore, to place a brief outline
of his experiments and views before the reader.

Just before falling asleep, and immediately before
becoming fully awake, many persons are subject to
hallucinations partaking of many of the characteristics
belonging to dreams. To them the name of hypna-
gogie (ὕπνος, sleep, and ἀγωγεύς, leader) hallucinations
has been given, i.e. hallucinations which lead to sleep.
Previous to M. Maury's investigations, the phenomena in question had attracted some attention from
German and French physiologists, but M. Maury's
investigations, many of which were performed upon
himself, throw more light upon the subject than it
has hitherto received.

According to M. Maury, the persons who most frequently experience these hypnagogic hallucinations
are those who are of an excitable constitution, and
are generally predisposed to hypertrophy of the
heart, pericarditis, and cerebral affections. This may
be true, but in two most remarkable instances which
have come under my observation, the type of organization was the very reverse of this.

In M. Maury's own case he finds that the hallucinations are more numerous and more vivid when he
experiences, as is frequent with him, a disposition to

---

* Le Sommeil et les Rêves; Études Psychologiques, etc. Troisième
édition. Paris, 1865.

cerebral congestion. Thus, when he has headache, nervous pains in the eyes, the ears, and the nose, and vertigo, the hallucinations make their appearance as soon as he closes his eyelids. Loss of sleep and severe intellectual exertions invariably produce them, as do also *café noir* and champagne, which, by causing headache and insomnia, strongly predispose him to the hypnagogic hallucinations. On the contrary, calmness of mind, rest, and country air lessen his liability to them. From the inquiries made of others by M. Maury, the results of his own experience, as well as from my own observations, I am well convinced that the hypnagogic hallucinations are directly the result of an increase in the amount of blood circulating through the brain rather than to actual congestion as he supposes. They therefore indicate the existence of a condition unfavorable to sound sleep. In the chapter devoted to the consideration of wakefulness the phenomena accompanying cerebral hyperæmia will be more fully considered.

The theory which M. Maury proposes in order to account for the existence of hypnagogic hallucinations further presupposes that as the power of the attention immediately before sleep begins to be diminished, and the mind cannot therefore voluntarily and logically arrange its thoughts, it abandons itself to the imagination, and that thus fancies arise and disappear unchecked by the other mental faculties. This absence of the attention need not be of long duration, a second, or even a shorter period being sufficient. Thus he lay down, and the attention which had been fully aroused soon became weakened; images appeared, and these partially reawakened the attention, and the current of his thoughts was resumed, to be replaced again by hallucinations, and this continued till he was fully asleep. As an example, he states that on the 30th of November, 1847, he was reading aloud the *Voyage dans la Russie Méridionale*, by M. Hommaire de Hell. He had just finished a line when he closed his eyes instinctively. In this short instant of sleep he saw hypnagogically, but with the rapidity of light, the figure of a man clothed in a brown robe, and with a hood on his head like a monk. The appearance of this image reminded him that he had shut his eyes and ceased reading. He immediately opened his eyelids and resumed his book. The interruption was practically nothing, for the person to whom he was reading did not perceive it.

M. Maury gives numerous examples of these hypnagogic hallucinations, all tending to show that they are induced by a congested condition of the cerebral vessels, and that thus, according to the views I have set forth relative to the condition of the brain in sleep, they are not to be regarded as precursors of that state, but of stupor.

In two very interesting cases of these hallucinations, which have come under my notice, they were brought about by any cause which increased the quantity of blood in the brain, or retarded the flow of blood from this organ. Thus, a glass of champagne, or a few 'drops of laudanum, would induce them, as also would the recumbent posture, with the head rather low.

As showing how readily dreams can be excited by impressions made upon the senses, M. Maury caused a series of experiments to be performed upon himself when asleep, which afforded very satisfactory results, and which are interesting in connection with the points already discussed in the present chapter.

1st Experiment. He caused himself to be tickled with a feather on the lips and inside of the nostrils. He dreamed that he was subjected to a horrible punishment. A mask of pitch was applied to his face, and then torn roughly off, taking with it the skin of his lips, nose, and face.

2d Experiment. A pair of tweezers was held at a little distance from his ear, and struck with a pair of scissors. He dreamed that he heard the ringing of bells; this was soon converted into the tocsin, and this suggested the days of June, 1848.

3d Experiment. A bottle of eau de Cologne was held to his nose. He dreamed that he was in a perfumer's shop. This excited visions of the East, and he dreamed that he was in Cairo in the shop of Jean Marie Farina. Many surprising adventures occurred to him there, the details of which were forgotten.

4th Experiment. A burning lucifer match was held close to his nostrils. He dreamed that he was at sea (the wind was blowing in through the windows), and that the magazine of the vessel blew up.

5th Experiment. He was slightly pinched on the nape of the neck. He dreamed that a blister was applied, and this recalled the recollection of a physician who had treated him in his infancy.

6th Experiment. A piece of red-hot iron was held close enough to him to communicate a slight sensation of heat. He dreamed that robbers had got into the house, and were forcing the inmates, by putting their feet to the fire, to reveal where their money was. The idea of the robber suggested that of the Duchess d'Abrantes, who he supposed had taken him for her secretary, and in whose memoirs he had read some account of bandits.

7th Experiment. The word *parafagaramus* was pronounced in his ear. He understood nothing, and awoke with the recollection of a very vague dream. The word *maman* was next used many times. He dreamed of different subjects, but heard a sound like the humming of bees. Several days after, the experiment was repeated with the words *Azor, Castor, Léonore.* On awaking, he recollected that he had heard the last two words, and had attributed them to one of the persons who had conversed with him in his dream.

Another experiment of the same kind showed like the others that it was the sound of the word and not the idea it conveyed which was perceived by the brain. Then the words *chandelle, haridelle,* were pronounced many times in rapid succession in his ear. He awoke suddenly, saying to himself, *c'est elle.* It was impossible for him to recall what idea he had attached to this dream.

8th Experiment. A drop of water was allowed to fall on his forehead. He dreamed that he was in Italy, that he was very warm, and that he was drinking the wine of Orvieto.

9th Experiment. A light, surrounded with a piece of red paper, was repeatedly placed before his eyes. He dreamed of a tempest and lightning, which suggested the remembrance of a storm he had encountered in the English Channel in going from Merlaix to Havre.

These observations are very instructive. They show conclusively that one very important class of our dreams is due to our bodily sensations. I have frequently performed analogous experiments on others, and had them practiced on myself, and have rarely failed in obtaining decided results. They strongly inculcate the truth of the conclusions arrived at in the foregoing chapter, and they serve as important data in enabling us to understand the division of the subject next to be considered.

In regard to the immediate cause of dreams the opinions of authors are very diverse. The older writers ascribe them to the rise of vapors from the stomach, to the visitation of demons, and other fanciful causes. Bishop Bull* declares that he knows

* Sermon on the Office of the Holy Angels toward the Faithful, quoted by Seafield. Op. cit , vol. i. p. 157.

from his own experience that dreams are to be ascribed "to the ministry of those invisible instruments of God's providence that guide and govern our affairs and concerns, viz., the angels of God;" and Bishop Ken held a similar view.

It would neither be possible nor profitable to refer at greater length to views which positive physiology has overturned. Observation and experiment have aided us greatly in arriving at definite conclusions on this subject, and the instances quoted on page 30 of this treatise, even if standing alone uncontradicted, would go far toward guiding us in the right path. On page 37 I have referred to the case of a man who, some time after receiving a severe injury of the head by which a considerable portion of the skull was lost, came under my professional care. Standing by his bedside one evening, just after he had gone to sleep, I observed the scalp slightly rise from the chasm in which it was deeply depressed. I was sure he was going to awake, but he did not, and very soon he became restless and agitated, while continuing to sleep. Presently he began to talk, and it was evident that he was dreaming. In a few minutes the scalp sank down to its ordinary level when he was asleep, and he became quiet. I called his wife's attention to the circumstance, and desired her to observe this condition thereafter when he slept. She subsequently informed me that she could always tell when he was dreaming from the appearance of the scalp.

My opinion, therefore, is that dreams are directly caused by an increased activity of the cerebral circulation over that which exists in profound sleep. This activity is probably sometimes local and at others general, and never equals that which prevails in the condition of wakefulness, when the functions of the brain are at their maximum of energy. This view is further supported by a consideration of the state of the brain in sleep and wakefulness, the condition of dreaming being, in a measure, an intermediate one. Illustrations of the effects produced by a notable increase in the quantity of blood circulating through the brain will be given in the chapter on wakefulness. All of these, it will be perceived, have a direct bearing on the question now under consideration.

CHAPTER VI.

MORBID DREAMS.

MORBID or pathological dreams are divided by Macario* into three classes: the prodromic, or those which precede diseases; the symptomatic, or those which occur in the course of diseases; and the essential, or those which constitute the main features of diseases. As this classification is natural and simple, I propose to follow it in the remarks I shall have to make on the subject.

PRODROMIC DREAMS.—There appears to be no doubt that diseases are sometimes preceded by dreams which indicate with more or less exactitude the character of the approaching morbid condition. Many instances of the kind which have been reported—especially by the earlier authors—are, however, in all probability merely coincidences; and in others the relation between the character of the dream and that of the disease is by no means clear.

Many cases of dreams indicating the nature of a malady which had not yet developed itself are referred to by Macario.† The instance of Galen's

---

* Op. cit., p. 86.   † Op. cit., p. 88, et seq.

(147)

patient, who dreamed that his leg had become converted into stone, and who was soon afterward paralyzed in that member, has already been cited.

The learned Conrad Gesner dreamed that he was bitten in the left side by a venomous serpent. In a short time a severe carbuncle appeared on the identical spot, and death ensued in five days.

M. Teste, formerly minister of justice and then of public works under Louis Philippe, and who finally died in the Conciergerie, dreamed three days before his death that he had had an attack of apoplexy. Three days afterward he died suddenly of that disease.

A young woman saw in a dream objects apparently confused and dim as through a thin cloud, and was immediately thereafter attacked with amblyopia, and threatened with loss of sight.

A woman, who had been under the care of M. Macario, dreamed at about the period of her menstrual flow that she spoke to a man who could not answer her, for the reason that he was dumb. On awaking she discovered that she had lost her voice.

Macario himself dreamed one night that he had a severe pain in his throat. On awaking he felt very well; but a few hours subsequently was attacked with severe tonsillitis.

Arnold, of Villanova, dreamed that a black cat bit him in the side. The next day a carbuncle appeared on the part bitten.

Dr. Forbes Winslow* gives several similar instances. A patient had, for several weeks before an attack of apoplexy, a series of frightful dreams, in one of which he imagined he was being scalped by Indians. Others dreamt of falling down precipices, and of being torn to pieces by wild beasts. One gentleman dreamed that his house was in flames, and that he was gradually being consumed to a cinder. This occurred a few days before an attack of inflammation of the brain. A person, prior to an attack of epilepsy, dreamt that he was severely lacerated by a tiger; and another, just before a seizure, dreamt that he was attacked by murderers, and that they were knocking out his brains with a hammer.

A barrister, for several years before an attack of cerebral paralysis, was in the habit of awaking from sleep in a condition of great alarm and terror without being able to explain the reason for his apprehension. Dr. Beddoes attended a patient whose first fit succeeded a dream of being crushed by an avalanche.

Gratiolet† cites additional examples. Thus, Roger d'Oxteryn, Knight of the Company of Donglas, went to bed in good health. Toward the middle of the night, he saw in a dream a man affected with the plague and entirely naked, who attacked him

---

* On Obscure Diseases of the Brain and Disorders of the Mind, etc., London, 1860, p. 611, et seq.

† Anatomie Comparée du Système Nerveux, etc. Par MM. Leuret et Gratiolet. Paris, 1839–1857, t. ii. 517, et seq.

with fury, threw him to the ground after a severe contest, and, holding him between his thighs, vomited into his mouth. Three days afterward he was seized with the plague and died. He also alludes to a case detailed by Gunther, in which a woman dreamt that she was being flogged with a whip, and on awaking found that she had marks on her body resembling the scars made by the lash.

The existence of diseases of the heart and larger vessels is often revealed by frightful dreams when there is no other evidence of their presence. Macario states that a young lady was under his care in whom violent palpitations of the heart were preceded by painful dreams. She subsequently died of disease of the heart.

Moreau (de la Sarthe),* in a very elaborate treatise on dreams, relates the case of a French nobleman, whom he had attended during several months for threatened chronic pericarditis, and who was at first tormented every night by painful and frightful dreams. These dreams, attracting attention, gave the earliest indication of the real condition, and excited fears as to the result, which were soon verified.

He cites another case in illustration of the fact that periodical hemorrhages are sometimes preceded by morbid dreams. A physician had, in his youth, been subject to periodical hemorrhages, but without dreams or other trouble during sleep. As he ad-

---

* Art. Rêves, in Grand Dictionnaire de Médecine.

vanced in years, the hemorrhages were not so frequent, but were always preceded by a condition of general irritation, characterized during wakefulness by heat of skin and frequency of the pulse, and during sleep by painful dreams. These dreams almost always related to violent actions, such as giving and receiving heavy blows, walking on a volcano, or being precipitated into lakes of fire.

Many cases of insanity being preceded by frightful dreams are on record. Falret,* in calling attention to the remarkable analogy which exists between mental alienation and dreams, says that it is an incontestable fact that insanity is often preceded by significant dreams, and that these constitute the whole essence of the disorder by becoming firmly fixed in the patient's mind. Thus, he relates that Odier of Geneva was consulted in 1778 by a lady, who, during the night preceding the outbreak of her insanity, dreamed that her step-mother approached her with a dagger in order to kill her. This dream made so strong an impression upon her that she ultimately accredited it as true, and thus became the victim of a delusion which rendered her a lunatic. He declares that numerous similar instances have come under his observation, and refers to the case of a young lady, subject to periodical attacks of mental derangement, whose paroxysms are always preceded by notable dreams.

---

* Des Maladies Mentales et des Asiles d'Aliénés, etc., Paris, 1864, p. 221.

Morel* affirms that many patients before becoming completely insane have frightful dreams, which they regard as evidences that they are about to lose their reason. Sometimes they are afraid to go to sleep on account of the terrifying apparitions which then visit them.

The following cases, related by Dr. Forbes Winslow,† are interesting in this connection:

"A gentleman, who had previously manifested no appreciable symptoms of mental disorder, or even of disturbed and anxious thought, retired to bed apparently in a sane state of mind. Upon arising in the morning, to the intense terror of his wife, he was found to have lost his senses! He exhibited his insanity by asserting that he was going to be tried for an offense which he could not clearly define, and of the nature of which he had no right conception. He declared that the officers of justice were in hot pursuit of him,—in fact, he maintained that they were actually in the house. He begged and implored his wife to protect him. He walked about the bed-room in a state of great agitation, apprehension, and alarm, stamping his feet, and wringing his hands in the wildest agony of despair. Upon inquiring into the history of the case, his wife said that she had not observed any symptoms that excited

---

* Traité des Maladies Mentales, Paris, 1860, p. 457.

† On Obscure Diseases of the Brain and Disorders of the Mind, etc., London, 1860, p. 614.

her suspicions as to the state of her husband's mind, but upon being questioned very closely, she admitted that during the previous night he appeared to have been under the influence of what she considered to be the nightmare, or a frightful dream. While apparently asleep he cried out several times, evidently in great distress of mind, 'Don't come near me!' 'Take them away!' 'Oh, save me; they are pursuing me!' It is singular that in this case the insanity which was clearly manifested in the morning appeared like *a continuation of the same character and train of perturbed thought that existed during his troubled sleep* when, according to the wife's account, he was evidently dreaming."

Dr. Winslow's second case is equally to the point: "I am indebted to a medical friend for the particulars of the following case. During the winter of 1849 he was called to see H. B., about five or six o'clock in the morning. The patient was the wife of a tailor and mother of three children. At this time she was rather emaciated and debilitated in bodily health, and anemic in appearance. She was of a religious turn of mind, and belonged to the Wesleyan persuasion. On the morning of the narrator's visit, he found the woman in a state of great mental excitement and under the influence of hallucinations. She had gone to bed apparently well, but during the night was the subject of a vivid dream, imagining that she saw her sister, long since dead and to whom she was much attached, suffering the pains of hell. When quite awake, no one could persuade her that she had been under the influence of an agitated dream. She stoutly persisted in maintaining the reality of her vision. During the whole of that day she was clearly insane; but on the following morning her mind appeared to have recovered its balance. She continued tolerably well, mentally, for four years, with the exception of her occasionally having moments of despondency arising from real or fancied troubles." * * *

The further particulars of this case, relating as they do to another division of the subject,—"sleep-drunkenness," as the Germans designate it,—will be considered under that head.

Without pretending to indorse all the conclusions of Albers,—as set forth in the following summary, and which I quote from a very learned and philosophical writer,*—there is no doubt that some of his dicta are well founded.

"Lively dreams are in general a sign of the excitement of nervous action.

"Soft dreams are a sign of slight irritation of the head; often in nervous fevers announcing the approach of a favorable crisis.

"Frightful dreams are a sign of determination of blood to the head.

---

* The Principles of Medical Psychology. Being the Outlines of a Course of Lectures, by Baron Ernst von Feuchtersleben, M.D. Sydenham Society Translation, p. 198.

"Dreams about fire are in women signs of an impending hemorrhage.

"Dreams about blood and red objects are signs of inflammatory conditions.

"Dreams about rain and water are often signs of diseased mucous membranes and dropsy.

"Dreams of distorted forms are frequently a sign of abdominal obstructions and diseases of the liver.

"Dreams in which the patient sees any part of the body especially suffering, indicate disease in that part.

"Dreams about death often precede apoplexy, which is connected with determination of blood to the head.

The nightmare (incubus ephialtes), with great sensitiveness, is a sign of determination of blood to the chest."

A very interesting paper on dreaming, by Dr. Thomas More Madden,* has been recently published, and from it I make the following extract:

"Intermittent fever is often announced, several days before any of the recognized symptoms set in, by persistent dreams of terrifying character. I have experienced this in my own person, and heard it confirmed by other sufferers on the African Coast. The following case of morbid dreaming ushering in yellow fever, I subjoin in the words of the gen-

---

* Medical Press and Circular; also Quarterly Journal of Psychological Medicine and Medical Jurisprudence, vol. i. p. 276.

tleman to whom it occurred, himself a medical man holding a high official position on the Gold Coast where it occurred.

" ' In the early part of 1840, I was an inmate of Cape Coast Castle, and as some repairs were then being made in the castle, the room assigned to me was that in which the ill-fated L. E. L. (Mrs. Maclean), the wife of the governor of Cape Coast, had been found dead, poisoned by prussic acid, not very long previously.   I had known her in London, and had been intimately acquainted with her history and much interested in it. Her body had been found on the floor near the door and in front of a window.   After a fatiguing excursion to some of the adjoining British settlements on the Coast, having retired to rest, I awoke disturbed by a dream of a very vivid character, in which I imagined that I saw the dead body of the lady who had died in that chamber lying on the floor before me   On awaking the image of the corpse kept possession of my imagination.   The moon was shining brightly into the part of the room where the body had been found, and there, as it seemed to me on awaking, it lay pale and lifeless as it appeared to me in my dream.

" 'After some minutes I started up, determined to approach the spot where the body seemed to be. I did so, not without terror, and walking over the very spot on which the moon was shining, the fact all at once became evident and obvious that no body was there—that I must have been dreaming of one.

I returned to bed, and had not long fallen asleep when the same vivid dream recurred; the same waking disturbance occurring while awake. As long as I lay gazing on the floor I could not dispossess my mind of that appalling vision ; but when I started up and stood erect it vanished at the first glance.

"'Again I returned to bed, dozed, dreamt again of poor L. E. L.'s lamentable end, and of her remains in the same spot; again awoke, and arose with the same strange results.

"' There was no more disturbance that night of which, at least, I was conscious, but when morning came fever was on me in unmistakable force in its worst form, and partial delirium set in the same night. I was reduced to the last extremity about the third or fourth night of my illness, when a conviction seized on my mind that it was absolutely essential to my life that I should not pass another night in Cape Coast Castle. I caused the negro servant I had fortunately brought out with me from England to have a litter prepared for me at dawn, and stretched on this litter, hardly able to lift hand or foot, I was carried out of my bed by four native soldiers, and was conveyed to the house of a merchant, and countryman of mine, to whose care and kindness I owe my life. So much for a visionary precursor of fever on the west coast of Africa.'

"In neuralgia, disturbed dreaming is occasionally a prominent symptom. In an obscure case I was

14

led to make what I believe to be a true diagnosis
from the indications furnished by the patient's
dreams. The individual in question is a man, aged
about 45, of an anemic habit, confined by a sedentary occupation, who, for many years, had suffered
from hemicrania, which lately had become more intense, and the intervals shorter. A couple of days
before the attack his sleep becomes broken by unpleasant dreams, and when the paroxysm has attained its height, he invariably dreams that he is the
helpless victim of a persecutor, who finishes a series
of torments by driving a stake through his skull.
During his recovery from each attack, he states that
his dreams are of a most agreeable character, though
so vague that he cannot give any account of them.
The frequent repetition of his dreams leads me to
conclude that there is some osseous growth within
the cranium, and that the vascular distention accompanying the neuralgic attack occasions pressure
upon this, giving rise to the sensation I have referred to, while the subsequent feeling of comfort
results from that pressure being removed."

A case has been recently published* in which the
dream immediately preceded, or perhaps even accompanied, the morbid action. A German, aged 45,
of a nervo-sanguineous temperament, went to bed
at 11 P. M., feeling as well as usual. Between 12

* Medical Investigator; also Quarterly Journal of Psychological
Medicine, etc., April, 1868, p. 405.

and 1 o'clock he dreamed that he saw his child lying at his side, dead. He was very much frightened, and at once awoke, to find that his tongue was paralyzed, and that he could not talk. The faculty of speech and the ability to move the tongue remained impaired for four months.

For several years past I have made inquiries of patients and others relative to their dreams, and have thus collected a large amount of material bearing upon the subject. With reference to the point under consideration, the data in my possession are exceedingly important and interesting. Among the cases which have come under my observation of diseases being preceded by morbid dreams, are the following:

A gentleman, two days before an attack of hemiplegia, dreamed that he was cut in two exactly down the mesial line, from the chin to the perineum. By some means union of the divided surfaces was obtained, but he could only move one side. On awaking, a little numbness existed in the side which he had dreamed was paralyzed. This soon passed off, and ceased to engage his attention. The following night he had a somewhat similar dream, and the next day, toward evening, was seized with the attack which rendered him hemiplegic.

Another dreamed one night that a man dressed in black and wearing a black mask came to him and struck him violently on the leg. He experienced no pain, however, and the man continued to beat him.

In the morning he felt nothing, with the exception of a slight headache. Nothing unusual was observed about the leg, and all went on well, until on the fifth day he had an apoplectic attack, accompanied with hemiplegia, including the leg which he had in his dream imagined to have been struck.

A lady, aged forty, who had been a great sufferer from rheumatism for many years, dreamt one afternoon, while sitting in her chair in front of the fire, that a boy threw a stone at her, which, striking her on the face, inflicted a very severe injury. The next day violent inflammation of the tissues around the facial nerve as it emerges from the stylo-mastoid foramen set in, and paralysis of the nerve followed, due to effusion of serum, thickening, and consequent pressure.

A young lady dreamt that she was seized by robbers and compelled to swallow melted lead. In the morning she felt as well as usual, but toward the middle of the day was attacked with severe tonsillitis.

A young man informed me that a day or two before being attacked with acute meningitis, he had dreamed that he was seized by banditti while traveling in Spain, and that they had taken his hair out by the roots, causing him great pain.

A lady of decided good sense had an epileptic seizure, which was preceded by a singular dream. She had gone to bed feeling somewhat fatigued with the labors of the day, which had consisted in attending three or four morning receptions, winding up with a dinner party. She had scarcely fallen asleep, when she dreamed that an old man clothed in black approached her, holding an iron crown of great weight in his hands. As he came nearer, she perceived that it was her father, who had been dead several years, but whose features she distinctly recollected. Holding the crown at arm's length, he said: "My daughter, during my lifetime I was forced to wear this crown; death relieved me of the burden, but it now descends to you." Saying which, he placed the crown on her head and disappeared gradually from her sight. Immediately she felt a great weight and an intense feeling of constriction in her head. To add to her distress, she imagined that the rim of the crown was studded on the inside with sharp points which wounded her forehead, so that the blood streamed down her face. She awoke with agitation, excited, but felt nothing uncomfortable. Looking at the clock on the mantle-piece, she found that she had been in bed exactly thirty-five minutes. She returned to bed and soon fell asleep, but was again awakened by a similar dream. This time the apparition reproached her for not being willing to wear the crown. She had been in bed this last time over three hours before awaking. Again she fell asleep, and again at broad daylight she was awakened by a like dream.

She now got up, took a bath, and proceeded to dress herself with her maid's assistance. Recalling

14*

the particulars of her dream, she recollected that she had heard her father say one day, that in his youth, while being in England, his native country, he had been subject to epileptic convulsions consequent on a fall from a tree, and that he had been cured by having the operation of trephining performed by a distinguished London surgeon.

Though by no means superstitious, the dreams made a deep impression upon her, and her sister, entering the room at the time, she proceeded to detail them to her. While thus engaged, she suddenly gave a loud scream, became unconscious, and fell upon the floor in a true epileptic convulsion. This paroxysm was not a very severe one. It was followed in about a week by another; and, strange to say, this was preceded as the other by a dream of her father placing an iron crown on her head and of pain being thereby produced. Since then several months have elapsed, and she has had no other attack, owing to the influence of the bromide of potassium which she continues to take.

In the case of a gentleman now under my treatment for epilepsy, the fits are invariably preceded by dreams of difficulties of the head, such as decapitation, hanging, perforation with an auger, etc.

A lady, previous to an attack of sciatica, dreamed that she had caught her foot in a spring-trap, and that before she could be freed it was necessary to amputate the member. The operation was performed; but as she was released, a large dog sprang at her and fastened his teeth in her thigh. She screamed aloud and awoke in her terror. Nothing unusual was perceived about the leg; but, on getting up in the morning, there was slight pain along the course of the sciatic nerve, and this before evening was developed into well-marked sciatica.

Insanity is frequently preceded by frightful dreams, and I have advanced several examples to this effect from the experience of others. We should naturally expect that very often the first manifestations of a diseased brain should appear during sleep. But dreams are of such a varied character, and so thoroughly irreconcilable with the normal mental phenomena of the wakeful state, that it is difficult to say that such or such a dream is evidence of a diseased mind. As, in some of the cases I have brought forward, a dream may take so firm a hold of the reason as to be the exciting cause of insanity, and not simply a sign of its approach, I am disposed, from my own experience, to regard the frequent repetition of the same dream as often indicative of a disordered mind, when very close observation would fail to reveal other evidences. There are, however, exceptions to this statement, as has been shown in the previous chapter.

Several cases, in which insanity was preceded by terrifying dreams, have come under my observation. In one of them a lady dreamed that she had committed murder, under circumstances of great atrocity. She cut up the dead body, but could not, with all her efforts, divide the head, which resisted her blows, with an axe and other instruments. Finally she filled the nose, eyes, and mouth with gunpowder, and applied a match. Instead of exploding, smoke issued slowly from the orifices of the skull, and was resolved into a human form, which turned out to be that of a police officer sent to arrest her. She was imprisoned, tried, and sentenced to execution, by being drowned in a lake of melted sulphur. While the preparations were being made for the punishment she awoke. She related the particulars of her dream to several friends, but it apparently made no great impression on her mind. The next night she dreamed of somewhat similar circumstances, and for several nights subsequently. On the sixth day, without any premonition, she attempted to kill herself by plunging a pair of scissors into her throat, and since that time to her death, which took place a few months subsequently, was constantly insane.

In this case there was no direct analogy between the character of her dream and the type of insanity which ensued. It cannot, therefore, be said that the dream produced the mental aberration. On the contrary, the dream was in all probability the first evidence of deranged cerebral action,—a condition which subsequently became developed into positive insanity.

The following case is similar to the foregoing in its general features:

A gentleman who had been unfortunate in some business speculations, shortly afterward became insane. Previous to this event he was troubled with frightful dreams, which gave him a great deal of annoyance, and frequently caused him to awake in terror. One of them occurred several times, and was of the following character. He dreamed that he was engaged to be married to a lady of beauty and wealth, and who was, moreover, possessed of great musical talent. One evening, as he in his dream was paying her a visit, she placed herself at the piano and began to sing. He remarked that he did not admire the piece of music she was singing, and asked her to sing something else. She indignantly refused. Angry words followed, and in the midst of the dispute she drew a dagger from her bosom and stabbed herself to the heart. As he rushed forward, horror-struck, to her assistance, her friends entered the room, and found him with the dagger in his hand. He was accused of murdering the lady, and, notwithstanding his protestations of innocence, was tried, found guilty, and sentenced to be hung. He always awoke at the point when preparations were being made for his execution.

A dream may make such a strong impression on the mind as to subsequently constitute the essential feature of the insane condition. This point has already been elucidated to some extent in the preceding pages. The following cases, however, are from my own records of practice.

A gentleman àwoke in the middle of the night, and, calling his wife, told her he had dreamed that a large fortune had been left him by a miner in California. He then went to sleep again, but in the morning again repeated the dream to his wife, and said that "there might be something in it." She laughed, and remarked that she "hoped it might prove true." About the time the California steamer was expected, the gentleman was observed to become very anxious and excited, and was continually talking of his expected fortune. At last the steamer arrived. He then began asking the postman for letters from California, went several times a day to the post-offiee to make like inquiries, and finally went aboard the steamer and questioned the officers on the same subject. Then he was sure the letter had miscarried, and would sit for hours in the most profound melancholy. He was now recognized by his family as a monomaniac, and strenuous efforts were made to cure him of his delusion, but they were unsuccessful; and although now apparently sane on other subjects, he still holds the erroneous idea which was first given him in his dream of several years ago.

A young lady was brought to me in July, 1868, who had been rendered insane by a dream which took place a few months before I saw her. She went to bed one night in good health and spirits, though somewhat fatigued in consequence of having skated a good deal the previous afternoon. In the morning she told her mother she had committed the "unpardonable sin," and that there was consequently no hope of her salvation. She based her idea on a dream she had had, in which an angel appeared to her, and sorrowfully informed her of her sin and her destiny. When asked to tell what her sin was, she refused to do so, saying it was too shocking and atrocious to talk about. She kept to her delusion, and soon settled into a sort of melancholic stupor, from which it was impossible entirely to rouse her. Under the use of arsenic, and the acid phosphate of lime of Prof. Horsford, she gradually recovered her reason.

The manner in which prodromic dreams are excited is very simple. The ancients and some modern writers have regarded them as prophetic; but the true explanation does not require so severe a tax on our powers of belief. In the previous chapter, it was shown that very slight impressions made upon the senses during sleep are exaggerated by the partially awakened brain. The first evidence of approaching paralysis may be a very minute degree of numbness—so minute that the brain when awake and engaged with the busy thoughts of active life fails to appreciate it. During sleep, however, the brain is quiescent, till some exciting cause sets it in uncontrollable action, and dreaming results. Such a cause may be the incipient numbness of a limb. A dream of its being turned into stone, or cut off, or violently struck, is the consequence. The disease goes on developing, and soon makes its presence unmistakable.

This explanation applies *mutatis mutandis* to all prodromic dreams. They are invariably based upon actual sensations, unless we except the rare cases which are simply coincidences.

SYMPTOMATIC DREAMS.—Morbid dreams are so generally met with in the course of disease, especially in that of the brain and nervous system, that I never examine a patient without questioning him closely on this point. The information thus obtained is always valuable, and sometimes constitutes the most important feature of the investigation.

Fevers are very often accompanied by frightful dreams. According to Moreau (de la Sarthe),* their occurrence indicates that the attack will be long, and that there is probably some organic affection present. My own experience agrees with that of Macario,† to the effect of not confirming these opinions. I have, however, generally observed that the frequency and intensity of the morbid dreams were in proportion to the severity of the fever.

Diseases of the heart are very generally attended with disagreeable dreams. They are usually short, and, as Macario remarks, relate to approaching death. The patient starts from sleep in terror, and sometimes it is difficult to convince him of the reality of his visions.

Dyspepsia and other diseases of the intestinal canal

* Op. cit., art. *Rêves*. † Op. cit., p. 95.

often give rise to morbid dreams. They are usually accompanied by a sense of impending suffocation, and ordinarily consist of frightful images, such as devils, demons, strange animals and the like. The presence of worms in the intestines is likewise a frequent cause of such dreams.

In *chlorosis* dreams are very common. Occasionally they are of a pleasant character, but in the majority of cases they are the reverse of this.

It would be difficult to mention a disease which is not, at some time or other of its career, an exciting cause of morbid dreams. The most interesting examples, however, are met with in cases of *insanity and other cerebral affections*, and frequently the delusions of the dreams are so mixed up with those which arise during the waking condition, that the patient is unable to separate them and to determine which are the consequence of erroneous sensations received when awake, and which are the results of dreams. The careful examination of almost any insane persons will also show that they incorporate the fancies of their dreams with the realities of everyday life. Indeed, the relations of dreaming to insanity are so interesting and important as to have attracted the marked attention of alienists and psychologists.

Cabanis* gives Cullen the credit of being the first

---

* Rapports du Physique et du Morale de l'Homme. Paris, 1824, tome second, p. 359.

15

to point out the 'similarity between the phenomena
of dreaming and those of delirium, and himself en-
ters at length into the full discussion of the several
questions involved. A very little reflection will suffice to convince the reader that the two conditions
are strikingly alike. In dreams we never distinguish
the false from the real; the judgment, if exercised at
all, acts in the most erratic manner; we are rarely
surprised at the occurrence of the most improbable
circumstances; our characters for the time being
often undergo a radical change, and we perform
imaginary acts in our sleep which are altogether at
variance with our actual dispositions. The hallucinations of sleep we accept as realities just as the insane individual believes in all the erroneous impressions made upon his senses. The dreaming person
is, in fact, the victim of delusions which, during the
existence of his condition, have a firm hold on his
mind and render him in no essential particular different from the one who suffers from mental un-
soundness. The incoherence present in dreams, and
the evident dependence of the various images upon
the suggestion of previous images, are likewise phenomena of the insane state.

Even in persons perfectly sane, dreams often produce a very powerful influence on the mind. Most
of us have, on awaking, felt pleased or disturbed
from reflecting upon the circumstances of a dream
we have had during the night, and occasionally the
impression has remained through the entire day.

With children this influence is still more strongly shown. As Sir Henry Holland* remarks, the corrections from reason and experience are less complete in them than in adults. As a consequence, they not infrequently confuse their dream-visions with the facts of their lives, and regard the former as real events. The hallucinations of dreams are also occasionally continued during wakefulness, and hence some persons have, on awaking, seen the images which had been present to them in their sleep.

The celebrated Benedict de Spinoza† was once the subject of an illusion which had its starting-point in a dream. He dreamed that he was visited by a tall, thin, and black Brazilian, diseased with the itch. He awoke, and thought he saw such an image standing beside him.

Muller,‡ in referring to such instances, says:

---

* Chapters on Mental Physiology. London, 1852, p. 126.

† B. D. S. Opera Posthuma, 1677, Epistola xxx. p. 471. In the course of this letter to his friend, Peter Balling, Spinoza says:

"Quum quodam mane, lucesente jam cælo, ex somnio gravissima evigilarem imagines, quæ mihi in somnio occurrerant, tam vividè ob oculos versabantur, ac si res finissent veræ, et præsertim cujusdam nigri et scabiosi Brasiliani, quem nunquam antea videram. Hæc imago partem maximam disparebat, quando, ut me alia re oblectarem, oculus in librum, vel aliud quid defigibam; quamprimium verò oculos à tali objecto rursus avertebam, sine attentione in aliquid oculos defigendo, mihi eadem ejusdem Æthiopis imago eâdem vividètate, et per vices apparebat, donec paulatim circa caput dispareret."

‡ Elements of Physiology, translated by Baly, vol. ii. p. 1394.

"I have myself also very frequently seen these phantasms, but am now less liable to them than formerly. It has become my custom when I perceive such images, immediately to open my eyes, and direct them upon the wall or surrounding objects. The images are then still visible, but quickly fade. They are seen whichever way the head is turned, but I have not observed that they moved with the eyes. The answers to the inquiries which I make every year of the students attending my lectures as to whether they have experienced anything of the kind, have convinced me that it is a phenomenon known to comparatively few persons. For among a hundred students, two or three only, and sometimes only one, have observed it. This rarity of the phenomena is, however, more apparent than real. I am satisfied that many persons would perceive these spectres if they learned to observe their sensations at the proper times. There are, however, undoubtedly many individuals to whom they never appear, and in my own case they now sometimes fail to show themselves for several months at a time, although in my youth they occurred frequently. Jean Paul recommended the watching of the phantasms which appear to the closed eyes as a means of inducing sleep."

If such phenomena take place in persons of healthy brains, the greater liability of the insane to experience them will readily be admitted.

The character of dreams, as Macario* remarks, varies according to the type of insanity to which the patient is subject. In melancholia they are ordinarily sad and depressing, and leave a deep and lasting impression; in expansive monomania they are gay and exciting; in mania they give evidence of the extraordinary mental excitement and activity of the subject, and in duration they are vague, fleeting, and occur but seldom.

ESSENTIAL MORBID DREAMS.—Under this head are comprehended the various forms of frightful dreams which are ordinarily designated under the name of nightmare. It has been my good fortune to have had the opportunity of carefully studying the phenomena of this singular affection in several persons of intelligence, and I propose, therefore, detailing the results of my own experience, after a short historical retrospect, which I hope will not prove uninteresting.

Nightmare is characterized by the existence during sleep of a condition of great uneasiness, the principal features of which are a sense of suffocation, a feeling of pain or of constriction in some part of the body, and a dream of a painful character. There are thus two essential elements of the affection—the bodily and the mental.

At a very early period the phenomena of nightmare attracted the attention of physicians. Hippo-

---

* Op. cit., p. 93.

15*

crates* describes it in the following words: "I have often seen persons in their sleep utter groans and cries, appear as if suffocated, and throw themselves wildly about until they finally waked. Then they were in their right minds, but were, nevertheless, pale and weak."

The general opinion held at that time was that the phenomena of nightmare were due to excess of bile and dryness of the blood. This view originated with Hippocrates, but was more or less modified by subsequent writers.

After the establishment of Christianity, the conviction began to prevail that during an attack of nightmare the subject was visited by a demon, who, for the time being, took possession of his body. Oribasius, in the fourth century, combated this idea, and endeavored to show that it was a severe disease, which, if not cured, might lead to apoplexy, mania, or epilepsy. He located it in the head.

Aetius also denied the existence of demoniacal agency in nightmare. He considered it as a prelude to epilepsy, mania, or paralysis.

During the middle ages nightmare was attributed to the power of the devil. Imps, male and female, called incubi and succubi respectively, were supposed to be the active agents in producing the affection. The treatment was in accordance with the theory, and consisted of prayers and exorcisms. Not unfre-

---

* Περὶ ἱερῆς νόσου.

quently the subject of the disease perished at the stake for the alleged crime of having sexual intercourse with incubi or succubi, according to sex.

Even in later times many persons have been found who believed implicitly in the reality of the visions which they experienced during an attack of nightmare. Thus Jansen* relates that a clergyman came to consult him. "Monsieur," said he, "if you do not help me I shall certainly go into a decline, as you see I am thin and pale,—in fact, I am only skin and bone; naturally I am robust, and of good appearance; now I am scarcely more than the shadow of a man."

"What is the matter with you?" said Jansen. "And to what do you attribute your disease?"

"I will tell you," answered the clergyman, "and you will assuredly be astonished at my story. Almost every night a woman, whose figure is not unknown to me, comes and throws herself on my breast, and embraces me with such power that I can scarcely breathe. I endeavor to cry out, but she stifles my voice, and the more I try the less successful I am. I can neither use my arms to defend myself, nor my legs to escape. She holds me bound and immovable."

"But," said the doctor, "what you relate is not in the least surprising. Your visitor is an imaginary

* Quoted from I. Franck by Macario, op. cit., p. 100.

being, a shade, a phantom, an effect of your imagination."

"Not so!" exclaimed the patient. "I call God to witness that I have seen with my own eyes the being of whom I speak, and I have touched her with my hands. I am awake, and in the full possession of my faculties, when I see this woman before me. I feel her as she attacks me, and I try to contend with her, but fear, anxiety, and languor prevent me. I have been to every one asking for aid to bear up against my horrible fate, and, among others, I have consulted an old woman, who has the reputation of being very skillful, and something of a sorceress. She directed me to urinate toward daylight, and to immediately cover the *pot de chambre* with the boot of my right foot. She assured me that on the very day I would do this the woman would pay me a visit.

"Although this seemed to me very ridiculous, and although my religion was altogether against my making any such experiment, I was finally induced, by reflecting on my sufferings, to follow the advice I had received. I did so, and, sure enough, on the same day the wicked woman who had so tormented me came to my apartment, complaining of a horrible pain in the bladder. All my entreaties and threats, however, were unavailing to induce her to cease her nocturnal visits."

Jansen at first could not turn this gentleman from his insane idea, but, finally, after two hours' conversation, he made him have some just conception of the nature of his disease, and inspired him with the hope of a cure.

Epidemics of nightmare have been noticed, and it likewise sometimes prevails endemically under certain peculiar forms. Thus vampirism, a belief in which exists in different parts of the world, is nothing but a kind of nightmare. Charles Nodier* gives some interesting details on this point, which I do not hesitate to transcribe.

In Morlachia there is scarcely a hamlet which has not several *vukodlacks* or vampires, and there are some, every family of 'which has its *vukodlack*, just as every Alpine family has its cretin. The cretin, however, has a physical infirmity, and with it a morbid state of the brain and nervous system, which destroys his reason, and prevents him appreciating his degraded condition. The *vukodlack*, on the contrary, appreciates all the horror of his morbid perception; he fears and detests it; he combats it with all his power; he has recourse to medicine, to prayers, to division of a muscle, to the amputation of a limb, and sometimes even to suicide. He demands that after his death his children shall pierce his heart with a spike, and fasten his corpse to the coffin, so that his dead body, in the sleep of death, may not be able to follow the instinct of the living body. The *vukodlack* is, moreover, often a man of note, often the chief of the tribe, the judge, or the poet.

---

* De quelques Phénomènes du Sommeil. Œuvres Complets, tome v. p. 170–175.

Through the sadness which is due to the recollection of his nocturnal life, the *vukodlack* exhibits the most generous and lovable traits of character. It is only during his sleep, when visited with his terrible dreams, that he is a monster, digging up the dead with his hands, feeding on their flesh, and waking those around him with his frightful cries.

The superstition is that during this state of morbid dreaming the soul of the sleeper quits the body to visit the cemeteries, and feast upon the remains of the recently dead.

In Dalmatia the belief is current that there are sorcerers whose delight is to tear out the hearts of lovers, and to cook and eat them. Nodier relates the story of a young man about to be married, who was the constant victim of nightmare, during which he dreamed that he was surrounded by these sorcerers, ready to pluck his heart from his breast, but who often awakened just as they were about to proceed to extremities. In order to be effectually relieved from their visitations, he was advised to avail himself of the company of an old priest, who had never previously heard of these horrible dreams, and who did not believe that God would give such power to the enemies of mankind. After using various forms of exorcism, the priest went peacefully to sleep in the same room with the patient whom he was commissioned to defend against the sorcerers. Hardly, however, had sleep descended upon his eyelids than he thought he saw the demons hovering

over the bed of his friend, alight, and, laughing hor-
ribly, throw themselves on his prostrate body, and
with their claws tear open his breast, and, seizing
his heart, devour it with frightful avidity. Unable
to move from his bed, or to utter a sound, he was
forced to witness this terrible scene. At last he
awoke to see no one but his companion, pale and
haggard, staggering toward him, and finally falling
dead at his feet.

These two men, adds Nodier, had had similar attacks. What the one dreamed he saw, the other
dreamed he had experienced.

As an instance of like dreams occurring to many
persons at the same time, the circumstances related
by Laurent* are worthy of notice.

"The first battalion of the regiment of Latour
d'Auvergne, of which I was Surgeon-major, while
in garrison at Palmi, in Calabria, received orders to
march at once to Tropea in order to oppose the landing from a fleet which threatened that part of the
country. It was in the month of June, and the
troops had to march about forty miles. They started
at midnight, and did not arrive at their destination
till seven o'clock in the evening, resting but little on
the way, and suffering much from the heat of the
sun. When they reached Tropea, they.found their
camp ready and their quarters prepared, but as the

* Grand Dictionnaire de Médecine, t. xxxiv., art. Incubi, par M.
Parent.

battalion had come from the farthest point, and was the last to arrive, they were assigned the worst barracks, and thus eight hundred men were lodged in a place which, in ordinary times, would not have sufficed for half their number. They were crowded together on straw placed on the bare ground, and being without covering, were not able to undress. The building in which they were placed was an old, abandoned abbey, and the inhabitants had predicted that the battalion would not be able to stay there all night in peace, as it was frequented by ghosts, which had disturbed other regiments quartered there. We laughed at their credulity; but what was our surprise to hear, about midnight, the most frightful cries issuing from every corner of the abbey, and to see the soldiers rushing terrified from the building. I questioned them in regard to the cause of their alarm, and all replied that the devil lived in the building; that they had seen him enter by an opening into their room, under the figure of a very large dog, with long black hair, and, throwing himself upon their chests for an instant, had disappeared through another opening in the opposite side of the apartment. We laughed at their consternation, and endeavored to prove to them that the phenomenon was due to a very simple and natural cause, and was only the effect of their imagination; but we failed to convince them, nor could we persuade them to return to their barracks. They passed the night scattered along the sea-shore, and in various parts of the town. In the morning I questioned anew the non-commissioned officers and some of the oldest soldiers. They assured me that they were not accessible to fear; that they did not believe in dreams or ghosts, but that they were fully persuaded they had not been deceived as to the reality of the events of the preceding night. They said they had not fallen asleep when the dog appeared, that they had obtained a good view of him, and that they were almost suffocated when he leaped on their breasts. We remained all day at Tropea, and the town being full of troops, we were forced to retain the same barracks, but we could not make the soldiers sleep in them again, without our promise that we would pass the night with them. I went there at half-past eleven with the commanding officer; the other officers were, more for curiosity's sake than anything else, distributed in the several rooms. We scarcely expected to witness a repetition of the events of the preceding night, for the soldiers had gone to sleep, reassured by the presence of their officers, who remained awake. But about one o'clock, in all the rooms at the same time, the cries of the previous night were repeated, and again the soldiers rushed out to escape the suffocating embrace of the big black dog. We had all remained awake, watching eagerly for what might happen, but, as may be supposed, we had seen nothing.

"The enemy's fleet having disappeared, we returned next day to Palmi. Since that event we have marched through the Kingdom of Naples in all directions and in all seasons, but the phenomena have never been reproduced. We are of opinion that the forced march which the troops had been obliged to make during a very hot day, by fatiguing the organs of respiration, had weakened the men, and consequently disposed them to experience these attacks of nightmare. The constrained position in which they were obliged to lie, the fact of their being undressed, and the bad air they were obliged to breathe, doubtless aided in the production."

A gentleman was, not long since, under my professional charge who was very subject to attacks of nightmare. Though remarkable for his personal courage, he confessed that during his paroxysms he was the most arrant coward in the world. Indeed, so powerful an impression had his frequent frightful dreams made upon him, that he was afraid to go to sleep, and would often pass the night engaged in some occupation calculated to keep him awake.

The dreams which he had were always of such a character as to inspire terror, and generally related to demons and strange animals, which seated themselves on his chest, and tried to tear open his throat. They came on a few minutes after he fell asleep, and lasted sometimes for more than an hour. During their continuance he remained perfectly still and quiet, giving no evidence of the tumult within, beyond the appearance of a cold sweat over the whole surface of the body. When he awoke, as he always did when the climax was reached, he started from the bed with a bound, and with all the evidences of intense fright. After that he was safe for the remainder of the night.

I am acquainted with another case in which there are no very obvious physical symptoms.

Ordinarily, however, the sufferer groans, and tosses about the bed; he appears to be endeavoring to speak, and to escape from his imaginary danger; his face, neck, and chest are flushed; a cold perspiration appears, especially on his forehead, and he is sometimes seized with a general trembling of the whole body. The respiration appears to be particularly disturbed; he gasps for air, and occasionally the breathing is stertorous. As to the pulse, strange as it may appear, there is rarely any marked change from the healthy standard, beyond the slight irregularity induced by the disorder of the respiration.

Among the mental symptoms, in addition to the fear with which he is filled, the sufferer is most sensibly impressed with a sense of his utter helplessness. His will is actively engaged in endeavoring to bring his muscles into action, but they cannot be made to obey its behests, and he consequently feels himself powerless to escape from the enemies which attack him.

In regard to the kind of images which make their appearance, there is more or less uniformity. Generally they consist of animals, such as hogs, dogs, monkeys, or nondescripts created by the imagination of the dreamer.· At other times they are demons of various forms. A gentleman, whose case came under my notice, was visited almost nightly by a huge black walrus, which appeared to roll off of a large cake of ice, and, crawling up the bed, to throw itself on his chest. Another was tormented by an animal, half lion and half monkey, which seemed to fasten its claws in his throat while seated on his breast.

At other times there are no images, but only painful delusions, in which the dreamer is placed in dangerous positions, or suffers some kind of torturing operation. Thus a lady informs me that she is subject to frequent attacks of nightmare, during which she imagines she is standing on the top of a high mast, and in extreme fear of falling off. Again she is dragged through a key-hole by some invisible power; and again has her nose and mouth so tightly closed that she can get no breath of air.

The *causes* of nightmare may be divided into the *exciting* and the *immediate*. The *exciting causes* are very numerous. Unusual fatigue, either of mind or of body, recent emotional disturbance, such as that produced by fright, anxiety, or anger, and intense mental excitement of any kind may produce it. I have known a young lady to have a severe attack the night after a school examination, in which she had been unduly tasked. Another young lady is sure to be attacked after witnessing a tragedy performed. A young man, who was under my care for a painful

nervous affection, always had a paroxysm of nightmare during the first sleep after delivering an address, which he was obliged to do every month for a
year or more.

Fullness of the stomach, or the eating of indigestible or highly stimulating food late in the evening,
will often cause nightmare. As Motet* remarks:
"One of the best-established causes is repletion of
the stomach, and slowness and difficulty of digestion.
Let an individual, habitually systematic, depart for
one day from the accustomed regularity of his meals,
let him change the hour of his dinner, and go to bed
before the work of digestion is completed, and it is
probable that his sleep will be troubled, and that
nightmare will be the consequence of his indiscre-
tion. · The painful feeling will be induced by distention of the stomach, by anxiety, and by the re-
straint given to the movements of the diaphragm."

Feculent food would appear to be especially powerful in causing nightmare, and according to Motet,
strong liquors and sparkling wines and coffee are
equally so. I have several times known it produced
by the New England dish of baked pork and beans,
and by green Indian-corn eaten just before going to
bed.

Various morbid affections, such as diseases of the

* Nouveau Dictionnaire de Médecine et de Chirurgie Pratiques,
tome sixième, Paris, 1867, art. Cauchemar.

heart, aneurism of the large arteries, affections of the brain or spinal cord, and diseases of the digestive or urinary apparatus are often exciting causes of nightmare. It may originate from painful sen sations in any part of the body. Some women, about the time of the menstrual flow, are particularly liable to paroxysms of this morbid dreaming.

Whatever interferes with the respiration or the easy flow of blood to and from the head may bring on an attack of nightmare. I have known it caused by the collar of the night-gown being too tight, and by the pillow being under the head and not under the shoulders, thus putting the head at such an angle with the body as to constrict the blood-vessels of the neck, and by the head falling over the side of the bed. I have not been able to ascertain that sleeping upon the back or on the left side predisposes to the affection, unless in those cases in which the former position causes snoring from relaxation of the soft palate.

The *immediate cause* of nightmare is undoubtedly the circulation of blood through the brain which has not been sufficiently aerated. The appearance of the sufferer is sufficient to indicate this, as the condition of the cerebral vessels and all the exciting causes act either by retarding the flow of the venous blood from the brain, or by impeding the respiratory movements. The effects of emotion, of mental fatigue, and of severe and long-continued muscular exertion are such that the nervous influence to the muscles of respiration is increased, or the muscles themselves are debilitated through this general fatigue of the organism. Fullness of the stomach acts mechanically, by interfering with the action of the diaphragm, and constriction about the neck directly increases the flow of blood through the brain. Certain diseases of the heart and lungs act upon the function of respiration, and thus interfere with the due oxygenation of the blood.

The *treatment* of morbid dreams presents no points of any difficulty. When they are the result of impressions made during sleep upon the nerves, and are the forerunners of disease, it is not very likely that physicians will be consulted as to their cure. Undoubtedly, however, much can be done to abate them when they belong to the category of prodromic dreams, as well as when they are symptomatic of existing disease. Hygienic measures, such as open-air exercise, attention to diet, and warm baths, and the use of the oxide of zinc and bromide of potassium, will do much to lessen the irritability of the nervous system, and to diminish any hyperæmic condition of the brain.

Nightmare often requires more active management, though even here we will ordinarily find the measures above mentioned the most effectual that can be taken for its treatment. Of course the exciting cause must be ascertained if possible, and means taken to remove it. This is not always an easy matter, and frequently cannot be accomplished without a considerable alteration in the course of life followed by the patient, and more or less sacrifice on his part. Among hygienic measures, I have several times found relief follow a sojourn at the seashore, and ocean bathing. Change of air is almost invariably beneficial, and moderate physical exercise, just to the point of fatigue, can scarcely be dispensed with. A gentleman, at this moment under my care, has been cured by a course of gymnastic training, which he took at my instance. The food of those subject to nightmare should always be plain, easily digestible, and moderate in quantity. Alcoholic beverages should always be sparingly taken, especially just before going to bed. Any article of food or drink known to produce the paroxysm, should of course be omitted altogether.

As to medicines, the whole round of so-called anti-spasmodics is usually tried by routine physicians. I have never seen them do any good. Iron and bitter tonics are indicated in cases of anæmia or exhaustion. As the disease is sometimes induced in children by the presence of worms in the alimentary canal, diligent inquiry should be made relative to symptoms indicating irritation from these parasites, and if they are found to exist, anthelmintics should be administered.

A case of intermittent nightmare, occurring every alternate night, in a young lady, was recently under my care. No exciting causes could be discovered, except the probable one of malaria. The affection yielded at once to the sulphate of quinia.

Ferrez* has published the details of a case of intermittent nightmare occurring in the person of a Spanish officer, who was attacked after passing forty-two nights at the bedside of a sick daughter. Every night, at the same hour, he was awakened by frightful dreams, which, irritating his brain, produced cramps, convulsive movements, an afflux of blood to the cerebral tissues, a sadness which he could not conquer, and a continual and powerful feeling of approaching death.

The patient, though of strong constitution, became enfeebled and emaciated. His countenance was pale, the pupils contracted, and his whole appearance showing the exhaustion consequent upon the battle which he was obliged continually to fight with his disease. He composed at this time some verses, describing in graphic terms the deplorable condition of his mind and body.

Gymnastics, temperance in eating and drinking, and the study of poetry, failed to give him relief. Finally he consulted Dr. Ferrez, who advised him to reveal his state to his family, who hitherto had been kept in ignorance of his malady, to continue his gymnastics moderately, not to eat in the evening, to drink only cold water, to use friction over the

---

* Gazette Médicale de Lyon, 15 Mai, 1856; also Macario, op. cit., p. 104.

whole surface of the body, to apply mustard plasters to the extremities, to sleep with his head elevated and uncovered, to bathe his head frequently during the night with cold water, to give up the study of poetry, and to devote himself to mathematics and political economy. These measures were rigorously carried out; but his daughter, who had been the involuntary cause of his disease, prescribed a better remedy than all the others. She had him waked at midnight, before the occurrence of his paroxysm, and thus broke up the habit.

Perhaps no one medicine is so uniformly successful in the ordinary forms of nightmare as the bromide of potassium, administered in doses of from twenty to forty grains, three times a day. I have seen a number of cases which had resisted all hygienic measures, and the simple removal of the apparent cause, yield to a few doses of this remedy.

When the affection has lasted a long time, it is more difficult to break up the acquired habit. In these cases, the plan so successfully employed by the daughter of the Spanish officer will almost invariably succeed.

Finally, persons subject to nightmare should so train the mind as to employ the intellectual faculties systematically, by engaging in some study requiring their full exercise. The action of the emotions should be as much as possible controlled, and the reading of sensational stories, or hearing sensational plays, should be discouraged. By severe mental training, individuals can do much to regulate the character of their dreams. It is a well-recognized fact, that intense thought upon subjects which require the highest degree of intellectual action is not favorable to the production of dreams of any kind.

CHAPTER VII.

SOMNAMBULISM.

THE phenomena exhibited by a person in the condition of somnambulism are so wonderful, that they have from the earliest times excited the superstitious feelings of the ignorant, and claimed the most serious attention of the learned. To see an individual apparently asleep to the greater part of surrounding objects, yet so keenly awake to others as to be able to perform the most intricate actions without the aid of the senses, is so greatly at variance with the common experience of mankind, as to call up feelings of astonishment, and perhaps of awe, in the minds both of the vulgar and those accustomed to scientific investigation. In those times, when the marvelous exercised so powerful an influence over mankind, and when all phenomena out of the ordinary course of everyday life were regarded as supernatural, it was the prevailing belief that the somnambulist was possessed. Modern science has at last dispelled this idea, and though it has not yet been able to furnish a rational theory of somnambulism which will account for all the manifestations of the affection, it has done much toward elucidating

(192)

the functions of different parts of the nervous system, and thus to prepare our minds for a full understanding of the subject.

Somnambulism has been defined* as "a condition in which certain senses and faculties are suppressed or rendered thoroughly impassive, while others prevail in most unwonted exaltation; in which an individual, though asleep, feels and acts most energetically, holding an anomalous species of communication with the external world, awake to objects of attention, and most profoundly torpid to things at the time indifferent; a condition respecting which most commonly the patient on awaking retains no recollection; but on any relapse into which, a train of thought and feeling related to and associated with the antecedent paroxysm will very often be developed."

This definition, though unnecessarily long and by no means perfect, will nevertheless suffice for a general description of the chief phenomena of the affection. It accords with the generally received theory. My own views of the nature of somnambulism will appear in the course of the following remarks.

In the introduction to his classical work on the subject under consideration, Bertrand† classifies the

* British and Foreign Medico-Chirurgical Review, April, 1845, vol. xix. p. 441.

† Traité du Somnambulisme et des différentes Modifications qu'il présente. Paris, 1823.

different kinds of somnambulism according to their causes. He recognizes—

1. A particular nervous temperament which predisposes individuals otherwise in good health to paroxysms of somnambulism during their ordinary sleep.

2. It is sometimes produced in the course of certain diseases, of which it may be considered a symptom or a crisis.

3. It is often seen in the course of the proceeding necessary to bring on the condition known as animal magnetism.

4. It may result as the consequence of a high degree of mental exaltation. It is in this case contagious by imitation to such persons as are submitted to the same influence.

From these four divisions of causes, Bertrand makes four kinds of somnambulism—the essential, the symptomatic, the artificial, and the ecstatic. As he wrote nearly twenty years before the publication of Mr. Braid's remarkable researches, he was of course unacquainted with that form of artificial somnambulism now known as hypnotism, and which may properly be included in his third class. I shall simplify his arrangement by dividing the several kinds of somnambulism into two classes—the natural and artificial.

Natural somnambulism may occur in persons who exhibit no marked deviations from the standard of health, and in whom there is no very evident nervous excitability. It is usually, though not always, manifested during ordinary sleep, and it is common for authors to speak of it as being necessarily connected with a dream. Thus, Macario* says it is a sleep in which the nervo-motor system and all the other organs are put in action under the influence of a dream. A few cases cited from other authors, and from my own experience, will tend to the more complete elucidation of the symptoms of this curious affection. Bertrand† quotes the following instance from the *Encyclopædia:*

" The Archbishop of Bordeaux has informed me that when at the seminary he was acquainted with a young ecclesiastic who was a somnambulist. Curious to ascertain the nature of the malady, he went every night to the chamber in which the young man slept. He saw, among other things, that the ecclesiastic got up, took paper, and composed and wrote sermons. When he had finished a page, he read it aloud—if one can apply the term to an action done without the aid of sight. When a word displeased him, he wrote the necessary corrections with great exactness. I have seen the beginning of one of his sermons which he wrote in the somnambulistic state, and thought it well composed and correctly written; but there was an alteration which surprised me. Having used the expression *ce divin enfant,* he thought as he read it over that he would change

---

* Op. cit., p. 117.　　　† Op. cit., p. 2.

the word *divin* for *adorable*.   He therefore effaced
the first word, and wrote the second above it.   He
then perceived that the word *ce* properly placed
before *divin* would not do before adorable; he therefore added a *t* to the preceding letters, so that the
expression read *cet adorable enfant*.   The same person, an eye-witness of these facts, in order to ascertain whether or not the somnambulist made use of
his eyes, put a card under his chin in such a manner
as to prevent his seeing the paper on the table; but
he still continued to write.   Wishing still to discover whether or not he distinguished different objects placed before him, the Archbishop took away
the paper on which he wrote and substituted several
other kinds at different times; but he always perceived the change because the pieces were of various
sizes.   When a piece exactly like his own was placed
before him he used it, and wrote his corrections on
the places corresponding to those on his own paper.
It was by this means that portions of his nocturnal
compositions were obtained. These the Archbishop
has had the goodness to send to me.   The most
astonishing among them was a piece of music written with great exactitude.   A cane had served him
for a ruler—the clef, the flats, and the sharps were all
in their right places.   All the notes were first made
as circles, and then those which required it were
blackened with ink.   The words were all written
below.   Once they were in such large characters
that they did not come directly under their proper

notes. He soon, however, perceived his error, and corrected it by effacing what he had written and writing it over again.

"One night, in the middle of winter, he imagined himself to be walking on the bank of a river and seeing a child fall in. The severity of the weather did not prevent him from determining to save it. He threw himself on his bed in the posture of a man swimming, went through all the motions, and, after becoming well fatigued with the severity of this exercise, he felt a bundle of the bedclothes, which he took to be the drowning child. He seized it with one hand, while he continued to swim with the other, in order to regain the bank of the imaginary river. Finally, he placed the bundle in a place which he evidently determined to be dry land, and rose, shivering, with his teeth chattering as though he had emerged from icy water. He remarked to the by-standers that he was frozen, that he would die of cold, and that his blood was like ice. He then asked for a glass of brandy in order to restore his vitality; but there being none at hand, a glass of water was given him instead. He, however, detected the difference and asked peremptorily for brandy—calling attention to the great danger he incurred from the cold. Some brandy was finally obtained. He drank it with much satisfaction, and remarked that he felt much better. Nevertheless, he did not awake, and, returning to bed, slept tranquilly the rest of the night."

Gassendi* had in his service a young man who every night arose in his sleep, descended into the cellar and drew some wine from a cask. Frequently he went out into the streets in the middle of the night, sometimes even he went into the country and walked on stilts, in order to cross a rapid stream which ran around the city. If he happened to awake from his sleep after having crossed this torrent, he was afraid to recross it so as to return home. Gassendi relates that when this man waked in the course of his perambulations he suddenly found himself in darkness, but as he had the faculty of remembering all that had taken place during his dream, and of recognizing the place where he found himself, he was able to grope his way to his bed. The darkness, therefore, which was an obstacle to the exercise of his sight when he was awake, was no impediment when he was in the state of somnambulism.

Dr. Prichard† cites from Muratori‡ the cases of Forari and Negretti, which are curious instances of the affection in question.

"Signor Augustin Forari was an Italian nobleman, dark, thin, melancholic, and cold-blooded, addicted to the study of the abstract sciences. His attacks occurred at the waning of the moon, and were stronger in the autumn and winter than in the

---

* Quoted by Bertrand, op. cit., p. 15.
† Cyclopædia of Practical Medicine. American edition, vol. iv. p. 196, article Somnambulism.
‡ Della Forza della Fantasia Umana. Venezia, 1766.

summer. An eye-witness, Vigneul Marville, gave the following description of them:

"One evening, toward the end of October, we played at various games after dinner; Signor Augustin took a part in them along with the rest of the company, and afterward retired to repose. At eleven o'clock, his servant told us that his master would walk that night, and that we might come and watch him. I examined him after some time with a candle in my hand. He was lying upon his back and sleeping with open, staring, unmoved eyes. We were told that this was a sure sign that he would walk in his sleep. I felt his hands and found them extremely cold, and his pulse beat so slowly that his blood appeared not to circulate. We played a tric-trac till the spectacle began. It was about midnight, when Signor Augustin drew aside the bed-curtains with violence, arose and put on his clothes. I went up to him and held the light under his eyes. He took no notice of it, although his eyes were open and staring. Before he put on his hat, he fastened on his sword-belt, which hung on the bedpost; his sword had been removed. Signor Augustin then went in and out of several rooms, approached the fire, warmed himself in an arm-chair, and went thence into a closet where he had his wardrobe. He sought something in it, put all the things into disorder, and, having set them right again, locked the door and put the key into his pocket. He went to the door of the chamber, opened it and stepped out

on the staircase.   When he came below, one of us
made a noise by accident; he appeared frightened,
and hastened his steps.   His servant desired us to
move softly and not to speak, or he would become
out of his mind; and sometimes he ran as if he were
pursued, if the least noise was made by those standing around him.   He then went into a large court
and to the stable, stroked his horse, bridled it, and
looked for the saddle to put on it.   As he did not
find it in the accustomed place, he appeared confused.   He then mounted his horse and galloped to
the house-door.   He found this shut, dismounted
and knocked with a stone, which he picked up, several times at the door.   After many unsuccessful
efforts, he remounted and led his horse to the water-
ing-place—which was at the other end of the court
—let him drink, tied him to a post and went quietly
to the house.   Upon hearing a noise, which the servants made in the kitchen, he listened attentively,
went to the door and held his ear to the keyhole.
After some time he went to the other side, and into
a parlor in which was a billiard-table.   He walked
around it several times and acted the motions of a
player.   He then went to a harpsichord, on which
he was accustomed to practice, and played a few
irregular airs.   After having moved about for two
hours, he went to his room and threw himself upon
his bed, clothed as he was, and the next morning
we found him in the same state; for as often as his
attack came on he slept afterward from eight to ten

hours. The servants declared that they could only put an end to his paroxysms either by tickling him on the soles of his feet, or by blowing a trumpet in his ears."

The history of Negretti was published separately by two physicians, Righellini and Pigatti, who were both eye-witnesses of the curious facts which they relate.

"Negretti was about twenty-four years old, was a sleep-walker from his eleventh year; but his attacks only occurred in the month of March, lasting at farthest till the month of April. He was a servant of the Marquis Luigi Sale. On the evening of the 16th of March, 1740, after going to sleep on a bench in the kitchen, he began first to talk, then walked about, went to the dining-room and spread a table for dinner, placed himself behind a chair with a plate in his hand as if waiting on his master. After waiting until he thought his master had dined, he removed the table, put away all the materials in a basket, which he locked in a cupboard. He afterward warmed a bed, locked up the house, and prepared for his nightly rest. Being then awakened, and asked if he remembered what he had been doing, he answered no. This, however, was not always; he often recollected what he had been doing. Pigatti says he would awake when water was thrown into his face, or when his eyes were forcibly opened. According to Maffei, he then remained sometimes faint and stupid. Righellini

assured Muratori that his eyes were firmly closed
during the paroxysm, and that when a candle was
put near to them, he took no notice of it. Sometimes he struck himself against the wall and even
hurt himself severely. Hence it would seem that
he was directed in his movements by habit, and had
no actual perception of external objects. This is
confirmed by the assurance that if anybody pushed
him, he got out of the way and moved his arms
rapidly about on every side; and that when he was
in a place of which he had no distinct knowledge,
he felt with his hands all the objects about him, and
displayed much inaccuracy in his proceedings; but
in places to which he was accustomed he was under
no confusion, but went through his business very
cleverly. Pigatti shut a door through which he had
just passed; he struck himself against it in returning. The writer last mentioned was confident that
Negretti could not see. He sometimes carried about
with him a candle, as if to give him light in his employment; but on a bottle being substituted, took it
and carried it, fancying that it was a candle. He
once said during his sleep that he must go and hold
a light to his master in his coach. Righellini followed him closely, and remarked that he stood still
at the corners of the streets with his torch in his
hand not lighted, and waited awhile in order that
the coach which he supposed to be following might
pass through the place where light was required.
On the eighteenth of March he went through nearly

the same process as before in laying a table, etc., and then went to the kitchen and sat down to supper. Signor Righellini observed bim, in company with many other cavalieri very curious to see him eat. At once he said, as recollecting himself, 'How can I so forget? To-day is Friday and I must not dine.' He then locked up everything and went to bed. On another occasion he ate several cakes of bread and some salad which he had just before demanded of the cook. He then went with a lighted candle into the cellar and drew wine, which he drank. All these acts he performed as usual, and carried a tray upon which were wineglasses and knives, turning obliquely when passing through a narrow doorway, but avoiding any accident."

Macario* cites from I. Franck the case of a young peasant, aged about sixteen, and endowed with a degree of intelligence above his age and condition, who was rendered somnambulic by the grief caused by the sudden death of his father. A few weeks after this event, he dreamed that he saw two unknown and frightful-looking men who advanced slowly toward his bed, and in menacing language ordered him to rise immediately and accompany them, threatening that if he refused they would return the following night and take him by force. This dream had so strong an effect upon him that he became melancholic. Two days afterward, while

---

* Op. cit., p. 127.

he was sleeping quietly, he dreamed that his father's spirit came to him, accompanied by the two men who had previously visited him, and ordered them to seize his son, notwithstanding his resistance, and to carry him off.

The young man dreamed that he was transported through a delightful country of vast extent; he heard the harmonious sounds from flutes and other musical instruments; he saw young people dancing on the charming plains, and he ate to satiety of delicious viands. Immediately the scene changed; his father's spirit disappeared, and his ferocious companions carried him high up into the air and then suddenly let him fall into a barrel. The servants returning with the cows, found the young man in the stable shut up in an empty barrel, scantily covered, and almost dead with cold and fright. Restored by frictions and warmth, he had no recollection of anything connected with his situation beside the dream above recorded. At the end of a week, he again rose from bed in his sleep, but finding the door locked, he returned and remained quiet. In a short time the disease ceased entirely.

The same author also quotes from Franck the case of a Jewish tailor, who, during the attacks of somnambulism to which he was subject, recited in a low voice his customary prayers in Hebrew. When he came to certain parts he raised his voice, called out aloud, and imitated the gestures of the rabbis in the synagogues. While thus engaged his eyes were wide open, and the pupils insensible to the stimulus of light. Then his face became pale, he presented the appearance of weeping, his whole body was covered with a cold, profuse sweat, and his pulse rose to 130. This crisis was followed by a tranquil prayer, to which sooner or later another access of fury succeeded; and this series continued for an hour or two, or till his prayers had been repeated for the prescribed period.

When strongly shaken he awoke with a startled manner, but if left to himself fell asleep again, and resumed his prayers at the place where he had been interrupted. When awake he declared that he had no recollection of what had happened during his sleep. The paroxysms appeared every day except Tuesday. The patient had a brother who was also a somnambulist.

These cases will give an idea of somnambulism as it has been witnessed by other observers, or as its phenomena have impressed them. The following instances of the disease have come under my own notice.

A young lady, of great personal attractions, had the misfortune to lose her mother by death from cholera. Several other members of the family suffered from the disease, she alone escaping, though almost worn out with fatigue, excitement, and grief. A year after these events, her father removed from the West to New York, bringing her with him and putting her at the head of his household. She had

not been long in New York, before she became affected with symptoms resembling those met with in
chorea. The muscles of the face were in almost
constant action, and though she had not altogether
lost the power to control them by her will, it was
difficult at times for her to do so. She soon began
to talk in her sleep, and finally was found one night
by her father, as he came home, endeavoring to open
the street-door. She was then, as he said, sound
asleep, and had to be violently shaken to be aroused.
After this she made the attempt every night to get
out of bed, but was generally prevented by a nurse
who slept in the same room with her, and who was
awakened by the noise she made in the room.

Her father now consulted me in regard to the
case, and invited me to the house in order to witness the somnambulic acts for myself. One night,
therefore, I went to his residence and waited for the
expected manifestations. The nurse had received
orders not to interfere with her charge on this occasion, unless it was evident that injury would result,
and to notify us of the beginning of the performance.

About twelve o'clock she came down stairs and
informed us that the young lady had risen from her
bed and was about to dress herself. I went up stairs,
accompanied by her father, and met her in the upper
hall partly dressed. She was walking very slowly
and deliberately, her head elevated, her eyes open,
her lips unclosed, and her hands hanging loosely by
her side. We stood aside to let her pass. Without

noticing us, she descended the stairs to the parlor, we following her. Taking a match, which she had brought with her from her own room, she rubbed it several times on the under side of the marble mantle-piece until it caught fire, and then, turning on the gas, lit it. She next threw herself into an armchair and looked fixedly toward a portrait of her mother which hung over the mantle-piece. While she was in this position, I carefully examined her countenance, and performed several experiments with the view of ascertaining the condition of the senses as to activity.

She was very pale, more so than was natural to her; here eyes were wide open and did not wink when the hand was brought suddenly in close proximity to them; the muscles of the face, which when she was awake were almost constantly in action, were now perfectly still; her pulse was regular in rhythm and force, and beat 82 per minute, and the respiration was uniform and slow.

I held a large book between her eyes and the picture she was apparently looking at, so that she could not possibly see it. She nevertheless continned to gaze in the same direction as if no obstacle were interposed. I then made several motions as if about to strike her in the face. She made no attempt to ward off the blows, nor did she give the slightest sign that she saw my actions. I touched the cornea of each eye with a lead-pencil I had in my hand, but even this did not make her close her eyelids. I was entirely satisfied that she did not see —at least with her eyes.

I held a lighted sulphur-match under her nose, so that she could not avoid inhaling the sulphurous acid gas which escaped. She gave no evidence of feeling any irritation. Cologne and other perfumes, and smelling-salts likewise failed to make any obvious impression on her olfactory nerves.

Through her partially opened mouth, I introduced a piece of bread soaked in lemon-juice. She evidently failed to perceive the sour taste. Another piece of bread, saturated with a solution of quinine, was equally ineffectual. The two pieces of bread remained in her mouth for a full minute, and were then chewed and swallowed.

She now arose from her chair and began to pace the room in an agitated manner; she wrung her hands, sobbed, and wept violently. While she was acting in this way, I struck two books together several times so as to make loud noises close to her ears. This failed to interrupt her.

I then took her by the hand and led her back to the chair in which she had previously been sitting. She made no resistance, but sat down quietly and soon became perfectly calm.

Scratching the back of her hand with a pin, pulling her hair, and pinching her face, appeared to excite no sensation.

I then took off her slippers, and tickled the soles of her feet. She at once drew them away, but no laughter was produced. As often as this experiment was repeated, the feet were drawn up. The spinal cord was therefore awake.

She had now been down stairs about twenty minutes. Desiring to awake her, I shook her by the shoulders quite violently for several seconds, without success. I then took her head between my hands and shook it. This proved effectual in a little while. She awoke suddenly, looked around her for an instant, as if endeavoring to comprehend her situation, and then burst into a fit of hysterical sobbing. When she recovered her equanimity, she had no recollection of anything that had passed, or of having had a dream of any kind.

A gentleman of very nervous temperament informs me that upon one occasion he dreamed that his place of business was on fire. He got up in his sleep, dressed himself, and walked a distance of over a mile to his store. He was aroused by the private watchman, who stopped him while in the act of looking through the grating of the door, under the impression at first that he had caught a burglar.

A young lady who some time since was under my care for intense periodical headaches, informed me that, just previous to each attack, she walked in her sleep, but had never any recollection of what she did while in the somnambulic state. Her mother stated that when her daughter was in this condition, she did not use her eyes, although they were wide

18*

open, nor did she appear to hear loud noises made close to her ears.

In relation to the activity of the senses during somnambulism, there is great diversity of opinion among those who have studied the affection. This is doubtless due to the fact that somnambulists differ among themselves as regards the use they make of their senses—some availing themselves of the aid they can derive from these sources, while others do not appear to employ them at all.

Thus it is stated that Negretti kept his eyes closed, and yet when a box of snuff was handed to him, he took a pinch without hesitation; and the young ecclesiastic whose case I have already quoted, performed even more complex acts than this

Castelli, a young somnambulist and a student of pharmacy, performed many astonishing acts during his paroxysms. One night he was found in the somnambulic condition, translating a passage from the Italian into French, and searching out the words in a dictionary. Prichard* assumes from this fact that he must have seen the words. He states further, that somnambulists have been known to write and even to correct their compositions, and to do other acts which could not possibly have been performed without sight. While it is certainly true that somnambulists have done all these things, it is equally

---

* Article Somnambulism, in the Cyclopædia of Practical Medicine, vol. iv. p 198, American edition.

certain that they have often performed them without the aid of their eyes. In the case of Castelli, a candle was on the table, which some one who saw him extinguished. He immediately arose, and lighted it, although there was no occasion for his doing so, as the room was well lit with other candles.* These he had not observed, but was only cognizant of the one which he probably did not see, but which was in relation with him through some more subtle channel.

Many somnambulists are known to have acted as though they saw in rooms which were perfectly dark. A gentleman informs me that his wife frequently walks in her sleep, and performs many somnambulic acts in entire darkness. On one occasion she went into a dark closet, and, opening a trunk, began to arrange the contents. It contained clothing of various kinds, which had been put into it the day before without being sorted. She classified all the articles, such as stockings, handkerchiefs, shirts, etc., without making a single mistake—and without the possibility of being assisted by light sufficient for ordinary eyesight.

Bertrand† refers to the case of a young lady who was accustomed to rise from her bed in a state of somnambulism and to write in complete darkness. A remarkable feature of this instance was, that if the least light, even that of the moon, entered the

---

* Bertrand, op. cit., p. 17.   † Op. cit., p. 18.

room, she was unable to write. She could only do so in the most perfect obscurity.

In the case of the young lady, the particulars of which, with my experiments, I have related, the sense of sight was certainly not employed, nor were the other senses awake to ordinary excitations.

On the other hand, it is evident that some somnambulists make use of their eyes and their other organs of sense in the ordinary way, when the excitations made upon them are in relation with the train of thought or ecstatic condition which prevails.

Macario,* in reference to this point, says:

"Somnambulists are insensible to external impressions, except those which are in relation with their ideas, their thoughts, and their feelings. It is thus that persons, the subjects of somnambulism, will pass before objects or individuals without seeing them, although they may have their eyes open. This phenomenon occurs often to individuals who are fully awake, although in a less degree. Thus when we are strongly preoccupied with any subject, the objects which surround us make no impression on our senses or our mind. Archimedes while meditating on a discovery, was an entire stranger to all that was going on around him. A part only of his brain was awake and active. While thus engaged, Syracuse was taken by the enemy, and he was not diverted from his thoughts either by the

---

* Op. cit , p. 132.

chant of victory by the conqueror, or by the cries and groans of the wounded and the dying."

As regards the sense of hearing, it is doubtless true that somnambulists rarely exercise it. There have been cases in which replies have been made to questions; but such answers have been given automatically, and not as if the mind took cognizance of the subject. A person intently engaged in reading, will often answer questions without suffering his train of thought to be interrupted. When he has ceased his study, he is surprised when told that he has been conversing.

The sense of taste appears to be very inactive in general, though in a few cases it has been manifested. The same is true in even a greater degree with the sense of smell.

The sense of touch is very differently affected, for so far from being diminished in its action, it is invariably unduly exalted. Though the eyes do not see, the ears hear, the tongue taste, or the nose smell, the somnambulist has one sense which is fully awake, and by which he is enabled to guide himself through the most devious passages in dangerous paths.

In this fact it appears to me we have a strong argument in favor of the theory of somnambulism which I have already referred to, and which appears to me to be supported by much additional evidence. I propose this view not without hesitation; but much study of the phenomena of somnambulism, and of analogous states of the nervous system, has certainly tended to convince me of its general correctness, and I am not without the hope that other students of neurology will find it reconcilable with their observations and experiments.

In my opinion, somnambulism is a condition of the organism in which through profound sleep the action of the encephalic ganglia is so materially lessened that the spinal cord becomes able to control and direct the body in its movements.

That the spinal cord even in the waking state constantly exercises this power, is a matter of common observation. I have already alluded to some of the facts which establish this proposition; but, for the purpose of giving as complete and connected a view as possible of all the points which bear upon the theory of somnambulism above enunciated, I shall not hesitate to recall them to the recollection of the reader, and to bring forward other circumstances which appear to be in relation with the question.

If an individual engaged in reading a book allows his mind to be diverted to some other subject than that of which he is reading, he continues to see the words, which make no impression upon his brain, and he turns over the leaf whenever he reaches the bottom of a page with as much regularity as though he comprehended every word he has read. He suddenly, perhaps, brings back his mind to the subject of his book, and then he finds that he has perused several pages without having received the slightest idea of their contents.

Again: when, for instance, we are walking in the street and thinking of some engrossing circumstance, we turn the right corners and find ourselves where we intended to go, without being able to recall any events connected with the act of getting there.

In such instances as these—and many others might be adduced—the brain has been occupied with a train of thought so deeply that it has taken no cognizance or superintendence of the actions of the body. The spinal cord has received the several sensorial impressions, and has furnished the nervous force necessary to the performance of the various physical acts concerned in turning over the leaves, avoiding obstacles, taking the right route, and stopping in front of the right door.

All cases of what are called "absence of mind" belong to the same category. Here the brain is completely preoccupied with a subject of absorbing interest, and does not take cognizance of the events which are transpiring around. An individual, for instance, is engaged in solving an abstruse mathematical problem. The whole power of the brain is taken up in this labor, and is not diverted by circumstances of minor importance. Whatever actions these circumstances may require, are performed through the force originating in the spinal cord.

The phenomena of reverie are similar in some

respects to those of somnambulism. In this condition the mind pursues a train of reasoning often of the most fanciful character, but yet so abstract and intense, that though actions may be performed by the body, they have no relation with the current of thought, but are essentially automatic, and made in obedience to sensorial impressions which are not perceived by the brain. Thus a person in a state of reverie will answer questions, obey commands involving a good deal of muscular action, and perform other complex acts, without disturbing the connection of his ideas. When the state of mental occupatiou has disappeared, there is no recollection of the acts which may have been performed. Memory resides in the brain and can only take cognizance of those things which make an impression on the mind, or of those ideas which originate in the encephalon.

In the case of a person performing on a piano, and at the same time carrying on a conversation, we have a most striking illustration of the diverse though harmonious action of the brain and spinal cord. Here the mind is engaged with ideas, and the spinal cord directs the manipulations necessary to the proper rendering of the musical compositiou. A person who is not proficient in the use of this instrument, cannot at the same time play and converse with ease, because the spinal cord has not yet acquired a sufficient degree of automatism, and the mind cannot be divided in its action.

Darwin gives a very striking example of the independent action of the brain and spinal cord. A young lady was playing on the piano a very difficult musical composition, which she performed with great skill and care, though she was observed to be agitated and preoccupied. When she had finished, she burst into tears. She had been intently watching the death-struggles of a favorite bird. Though her brain was thus absorbed, the spinal cord had not been diverted from the office of carrying on the muscular and automatic actions required by her musical performance.

The brain cannot entertain two ideas or initiate two acts at the same time. A person cannot, for example, think of a lamp and a book simultaneously; the thought of the one and the thought of the other will be found to alternate by any one who feels inclined to make the experiment, and not to exist at the same time. Neither can the brain think and simultaneously will. Whatever volitional acts it performs, are distinct from thought, and clearly separated from it by the element of time.

Now in all sleep there is more or less somnambulism, because the brain, according as the sleep is more or less profound, is more or less removed from the sphere of action. If this quiescent state of the brain is accompanied, as it frequently is in nervous and excitable persons, by an exalted condition of the spinal cord, we have the higher order of somnambulic phenomena produced, such as walking and the performance of complex and apparently syste-

matic movements; if the sleep of the brain be somewhat less profound, and the spinal cord less excitable, the somnambulic manifestations do not extend
beyond sleep-talking; a still less degree of cerebral
inaction and spinal irritability produces simply a
restless sleep and a little muttering; and when the
sleep is perfectly natural, and the nervous system of
the individual well balanced, the movements do not
extend beyond changing the position of the head
and limbs and turning over in bed.

As regards the power of the spinal cord to supply
the nervous force requisite for the performance of
such actions as those specified, I do not think there
can be any question. Much observation and many
experiments have convinced me that the importance of the spinal cord as a center of intellection
and volition has been unwarrantably ignored. It is
of course not a matter for doubt that the faculty of
consciousness is latent in the spinal cord so long as
the brain is in a state of activity, and that the faculty
of memory does not reside in it at all. When the
brain acts, it ordinarily assumes the control of the
cord; but there are times, especially during the
course of certain diseases, when the latter obtains
the mastery over the superior organ and dominates
with terrible power.

The actions initiated by the spinal cord are more
or less automatic in their character—though not
altogether so. The motions of a frog deprived of
its brain, show a certain amount of intellection and

volition. That they are not more extensive is probably due to the fact that all the organs of the senses,
except that of touch, have been removed with the
brain. In persons engaged in intense thought and
performing actions not in accordance therewith, the
impressions made upon the organs of the senses are
not appreciated by the brain, but pass through its
substance to the spinal cord with which they are in
connection by continuity of structure, and which
initiates the subsequent actions.

In the somnambulic individual the brain is still
more incapable of receiving sensorial impressions.
Whatever sense is therefore exercised during the
condition of somnambulism, owes its activity to the
spinal cord; but in most cases of the state in question, the brain is so profoundly asleep that it does
not even transmit impressions to the cord, and hence
there are no sensations at all, except that of touch,
unless the irritations capable of exciting them are
extraordinarily great.

In artificial somnambulism—the hypnotism of
Braid—the spinal cord acquires a very high degree
of susceptibility to sensorial impressions, and the
brain is even more incapable than in natural somnambulism of asserting its superiority. But the
consideration of this interesting branch of the subject does not enter into the plan of the present work.

The *causes* of somnambulism are generally to be
found inherent in the organism of the individual,
though they may be excited to activity by many

circumstances which are capable of exhausting the nervous system or producing emotional disturbance. Young persons are more subject than those of maturer age, and there are few children who do not exhibit at some time or other manifestations of the condition in question, such as muttering and talking in their sleep, laughing, crying, or getting out of bed. Persons of the nervous temperament are those most liable to be affected. In four cases of chorea which have come under my care, the subjects were sleep-walkers in their youth, and the young lady whose case I have related was choreic at the time.

In regard to the *treatment* there is not much to be said. In the great majority of cases the affection yields readily to appropriate measures; the most efficacious of which consists in means adapted to break up the habit. This may be done by waking the patient before the expected paroxysm, or by placing a tub of cold water so that the feet will be put into it on the attempt to leave the bed. Full exercise in the open air, the avoidance of luxurious habits, and sleeping with the head well raised, are always beneficial.

Of medicines, I have no experience except with the bromide of potassium, and those calculated to improve the tone of the nervous system. The former I have used in two cases with entire success. One of them was that of the young lady, the details of whose case I have related; the other that of a gentleman, forty years of age, who became somnambulic from mental excitement, due to the extensive business operations in which he was engaged. Large doses of this remedy—forty to sixty grains taken at bedtime, and smaller doses, ten to thirty grains, taken twice through the day—broke up the habit entirely in a few weeks. Among the other remedies, I have employed phosphorus, strychnia, and iron with manifest advantage. Cold baths are generally useful. I am acquainted with a young lady who cured herself by taking a cold bath every night just before going to bed. The so-called antispasmodics can scarcely be useful.

Much may be done also by suitable mental training. The reading of exciting fictions, and the witnessing of sensational theatrical exhibitions, are always prejudicial to persons subject to attacks of somnambulism.

CHAPTER VIII.

THE PATHOLOGY OF WAKEFULNESS.

As nations advance in civilization and refinement, affections of the nervous system become more frequent, because progress in these directions is necessarily accompanied by an increase in the wear and tear of those organs through which perceptions are received and emotions excited; and, in addition, the mode of life, as regards food, clothing, occupation, and habits, is being constantly removed farther from that standard which a regard for hygienic considerations would establish as most advantageous. If, as we have every reason to believe, each thought involves the destruction of a certain amount of nervous tissue, we can very well understand why, as we go forward in enlightenment and in all the elements of material and intellectual progress, we are at the same time, unless we also advance in the knowledge of the laws of our being, hurrying ourselves with rapid strides to a state of existence in which there is neither waste nor repair.

I am far, however, from desiring to be understood as intimating that a high state of civilization is antagonistic to long life or health. What is lost in

(222)

these directions as regards the nervous system is more than made up by the increased provision afforded for comfort in other ways. But while we have improved the hygienic condition of our cities and dwellings; while we as a rule clothe our bodies according to the principles of sanitary science and common sense; and while cleanliness of person has become the rule, and filthiness the exception, we have made little or no progress in the hygienic management of those organs which place us in relation with the world, and a healthy condition of which is so essential to our happiness.

Among the many derangements in the normal operation of the nervous system, induced by irregular or excessive cerebral action, those which relate to the function of sleep are certainly not the least in importance, whether regard be had to the actual comfort of the individual or to the serious consequences to which they may give rise. To the consideration of some of these morbid conditions I propose to devote the remainder of the present volume, and first to inquire into the most important of them, wakefulness or insomnia.

As a symptom of various diseases which affect the human organism, wakefulness is sufficiently well recognized by systematic writers on the practice of medicine, though, even here, it is very certain that its pathology has seldom been clearly made out. As a functional disorder of the brain, arising from inordinate mental activity, it has received scarcely any notice. This neglect has, doubtless, been in a great measure due to the fact that it is only within late years that the condition in question has become so common as to attract much attention. At present there are, probably, but few physicians engaged in extensive practice in any of our large cities who do not in the course of the year meet with several cases of obstinate wakefulness, unaccompanied, in the early stages at least, by any other prominent disorder of the system.

In my opinion, no one cause is so productive of cerebral affections as persistent wakefulness, for not only is the brain prevented from obtaining rest, but it is kept in a state of erethism, which, if not relieved, must sooner or later end in organic disease. Southey laid the seeds of that disorder which terminated in the loss of his intellect, by watching at the bedside of his sick wife during the night, after the excessive literary labors of the day.* Newton's mind also suffered in the later years of his life through deprivation of sleep;† and Dr. Forbes Winslow, in remarking on Southey's case, says: "No brain can remain in permanent health that has been overtasked by nightly vigils still more than by daily labor."‡

---

* The Scenery and Poetry of the English Lakes. By Charles Mackay, LL.D.

† Life of Sir Isaac Newton. By Sir David Brewster, vol ii. p. 240.

‡ On Obscure Diseases of the Brain, etc. London, 1860, p. 609.

Renaudin,* in a very philosophical essay, calls attention to the fact that persistent wakefulness is sooner or later followed by insanity; and Maury† states his opinion to the same effect. The remarks of Dr. Ray‡ upon this subject are so apposite that I reproduce them in part, commending at the same time the little book from which they are taken to the attention of the reader.

"A periodical renewal of the nervous energies as often as once a day is an institution of nature, none the less necessary to the well-being of the animal economy, because in some degree under the control of the will. To disregard its requirements with impunity is no more possible than it is to violate any other organic law with impunity, and no man need flatter himself that he may systematically intrench upon the hours usually devoted to rest and still retain the freshness and elasticity of his faculties. With the same kindliness that marks all the arrangements of the animal economy, this condition is attended with many pleasing sensations and salutary effects, gently alluring us to seek the renovation which it offers. 'While I am asleep,' says the immortal Sancho Panza, 'I have neither fear nor hope; neither trouble nor glory; and blessings on

---

* Sur l'Influence Pathologique de l'Insomnie. Annales Médico-Psychologiques, 3me Série, t. iii. p. 384, et seq.

† Le Sommeil et les Rêves. 3me éd. Paris, 1865, p. 9.

‡ Mental Hygiene. Boston, 1863, p. 97.

him who invented sleep,—the mantle that covers all human thoughts; the food that appeases hunger; the drink that quenches thirst; the fire that warms; the cold that moderates heat; and, lastly, the general coin that purchases all things; the balance and weight that make the shepherd equal to the king and the simple to the wise.' The ill effects of iusufficient sleep may be witnessed on some of the principal organic functions, but it is the brain and nervous system that suffer chiefly and in the first instance. The consequences of a too protracted vigil are too well known to be mistaken, and many a person is suffering, unconscious of the cause, from the habit of irregular and insufficient sleep. One of its most common effects is a degree of nervous irritability and peevishness, which even the happiest self-discipline can scarcely control. That buoyancy of the feelings, that cheerful, hopeful, trusting temper that springs far more from organic conditions than from mature and definite convictions, give way to a spirit of dissatisfaction and dejection; while the even demeanor, the measured activity, are replaced either by a lassitude that renders any exertion painful, or an impatience and restlessness not very conducive to happiness. Upon the intellectual powers the mischief is still more serious. They not only lose that healthy activity which combines and regulates their movements in the happiest manner, but they are no longer capable of movements, once perfectly easy. The conceptions cease to be clear and well defined, the power of endurance is weakened, inward perceptions are confounded with outward unhappiness, and illusory images obtrude themselves unbidden upon the mind. This kind of disturbance may pass sooner or later into actual insanity, and many a noble spirit has been utterly prostrated by habitual loss of rest."

CASE I.—Some years ago a case similar in several respects to that of Southey came under my observation. A gentleman of superior mind and of great powers of application spent from sixteen to eighteen hours each day in severe literary labor. This of itself would have been a heavy strain to most persons, but he went regularly to bed and slept soundly six hours each night, and it is possible that he might have continued this mode of life for several years without serious inconvenience, when his wife was suddenly taken ill. His anxiety on her account was very great, and he spent nearly the whole night by her bedside, sleeping only for about an hour toward morning. After three weeks passed in this manner, his wife was pronounced out of danger, but he found it impossible to resume his former habits. He could neither study nor sleep. The nights were passed in walking the floor of his chamber or in tossing restlessly on his bed. There were no pain, no fever, no disorder of any other organ. There was nothing but ceaseless activity of the mind and an utter inability to sleep. Stimulants and narcotics only increased the violence of his symptoms, and every other means employed failed to give relief. The danger of his situation was pointed out to him and travel recommended. He followed the advice, and though it was several months before he was completely relieved, his condition began at once to improve. He was taught a lesson which has not been without influence, in causing him to task his mental faculties less severely.

CASE II.—Another, an intimate friend, who occupied an important public position, gave so much time and attention to his duties, which were of a highly laborious character, that be deprived himself of the amount of sleep to which he had previously been accustomed. It was rarely the case that he got to bed before two or three o'clock in the morning, and then an hour or two was always occupied in active intellection. The consequence was that he finally broke down through want of the mental repose so essential to him. Inflammation of the brain ensued, and this terminated in acute insanity, from which he died.

It would be easy to bring forward other instances of which I am perfectly cognizant, or which have been cited by authors in illustration of the point in question, but it is scarcely necessary to enlarge further upon this portion of the subject. We should be careful, however, not to mistake the effect for the cause, an error which is often committed in this as well as in other matters. It is well known that many cases of insanity are marked in the early stages by persistent insomnia. Doubtless this is frequently a consequence of the morbid action already set up in the brain; but much observation has satisfied me that it is more often the cause of the cerebral aberration, and that by proper medical treatment the mental excitement may be generally allayed. Certainly the means most commonly resorted to in such instances are adopted without the full consideration so imperatively necessary, and consequently are fully as liable to increase as to lessen the disturbance.

We cannot employ too much care in doing everything in our power to prevent the occurrence of those slight attacks of cerebral congestion, which, though perhaps scarcely observable at the time, are yet fraught with very serious consequences. Persons have had their whole characters changed by an apparently trifling interference with the circulation of blood in the head. A person of my acquaintance was naturally of good disposition, amiable in his character, and considerate in his dealings with others; but after an attack of vertigo, attended with unconsciousness of but a few moments' duration, his whole mental organization underwent a radical change. He became deceitful, morose, and exceedingly overbearing and tyrannical toward all with whom he came in contact, and whom it was safe for him to maltreat. Tuke and Bucknill* refer to the

* A Manual of Psychological Medicine, etc. London, 1858, p. 375.

case of a lady whose character had always been distinguished for conscientiousness, whose religious education had been of a somber kind, and who, suffering under an attack of small-pox attended with congestion of the brain, recovered, with the natural bent of her disposition greatly exaggerated. The irritability of conscience had become an actual disease, destroying the happiness of the individual and rendering her incompetent to discharge any of the duties of life. The same authors also mention the instance of a distinguished admiral who had always been remarkable for pride and liability to passionate anger, becoming the subject of cerebral excitement, loss of sleep, and general feverishness consequent upon the chagrin caused by a supposed neglect by the government.

In primary insomnia there is always an increase in the quantity of blood circulating in the brain. This is either absolute or relative. The former is the case when there has been no exhausting disease, hemorrhage, or other debilitating influence in operation, and while, though general good health exists, the amount of blood in the cranium is augmented; the latter, when from any cause the system has become reduced, and when, while this condition prevails, a temporary activity takes place in the cerebral circulation. The first may properly be called active, the latter passive insomnia. In the one there is more blood in the brain than is normally present; in the other, though there may be less blood than in health, the quantity is increased over the amount to which the brain has in a measure accustomed itself.

Thus if we suppose the cerebral vessels of a healthy brain to contain ordinarily a pint of blood, and the amount to be increased to a pint and a half, and continued at this standard for several consecutive days, a state of active insomnia ensues. If, on the other hand, this pint should be reduced to a gill by any cause producing general debility, such as hemorrhage, starvation, or disease, and then by some exciting mental emotion, the excessive use of alcoholic liquors, or other influence acting for a considerable period, be increased to half a pint, a condition of passive insomnia would be produced— the latter condition resulting not from a disturbance of the normal relation existing between the *intra* and *extra* cranial blood, but of that which has been established by morbific causes, and to which the organism has become habituated.

CASE IH.—The following is a good example of the active form of morbid wakefulness:

A short time since a gentleman was under my charge in whose case the only deviation from health which could be perceived was an utter inability to sleep. Being by profession a broker, and passing his days, and a great portion of his nights, in the stock and gold rooms, during a period of great financial excitement, his brain had been kept so continually in a state of intense action that it was impossible for him, when he went to bed, to compose his mind so as to allow of sleep ensuing. Thoughts similar to those which were excited during his business operations were in full flow, notwithstanding all his efforts to banish them. Calculations were entered into, and speculations were constantly being formed with as great or even greater facility than during the day. Many of the latter were of the most extravagant character, a fact of which he was fully aware at the time, but he nevertheless found it impossible to refrain from indulging in them. All his other functions were performed with regularity. His appetite was good, he took a not inconsiderable amount of exercise, and he committed no excesses of any kind except as regarded his brain. When I first saw him he had not slept for six nights, although he had taken large quantities of brandy, morphine, and laudanum; but beyond a slight feeling of confusion in his mind at times, and a little pain in his eyeballs, he experienced no unpleasant sensations during the day. As soon, however, as his head touched the pillow, and he tried to get to sleep, a feeling of the most intense uneasiness came over him, while at the same time his face and ears became hot and flushed. His mental faculties were roused into increased action; he tossed restlessly from one side of the bed to the other, and by the time morning came he was thoroughly exhausted, mentally and physically. A cold bath and a breakfast of two large cups of coffee, beefsteak and eggs, set him up for the balance of the day, till he retired to bed, when the phenomena of the previous night would be repeated.

In this case I conceived that the blood-vessels of the brain, from overdistention, had lost, in a great measure, their contractile power, and that a larger quantity of blood was, in consequence, circulating within the cranium than was normal. The vessels were therefore in a condition very similar to that of a bladder in which, from the desire to urinate having been too long resisted, contraction cannot be induced even by the most strenuous exertion of the will. As the gentleman was of strong, athletic build, and otherwise in full health, blood-letting would undoubtedly have proved of great service; but, for reasons which will appear hereafter, I determined to try a remedy less likely to do harm, and fully as capable of doing good. I administered thirty grains of the bromide of potassium at six o'clock in the evening, and repeated the dose at ten, directing him to go to bed half an hour subsequently. The first dose produced a decided sedative action, and the second was still more effectual in calming the mental excitement. When he lay down, his mind was not disturbed by a flow of thoughts, and he fell almost unconsciously into a quiet sleep, from which he did not awake till near seven o'clock the following morning. There were no unpleasant symptoms of any kind; on the contrary, he felt strengthened and refreshed. The next night one dose was ad-

ministered at about bedtime, which was also followed by a sound and invigorating sleep. No further treatment was given, as on the following night
sleep came naturally.

Sir Benjamin Brodie,* without, however, making
the distinction I have insisted upon, refers to the
active or sthenic type of wakefulness in the following quotations from a little work which should be
in the hands of all who are interested in the philosophy of the mind.

Speaking of the causes of the wakefulness of some
persons, he savs: "At the same time there is no
doubt that there is sometimes a morbid condition
of the nervous system, the nature of which we
cannot well explain, which is incompatible with
sleep. The patient says, 'I feel fatigued and wearied
and want to go to sleep, but I cannot sleep.'"

In asserting as he does that this kind of wakefulness is sometimes the forerunner of mental derangement, Sir Benjamin is supported by many cases detailed by authors on psychological medicine, and
the following, which he gives,† is directly to the
point:

"A gentleman of my acquaintance in whose
family circumstances had occurred which were to
him sources of intense anxiety, passed six entire
days and nights without sleep. At the end of this

* Psychological Inquiries. Third edition, London, 1856, p. 141.
† Op. cit. p. 142.

time he became affected with illusions of such a
nature that it was necessary to place him in confinement. After some time he recovered perfectly.
He had never shown any signs of mental derangement before, nor has any one of his family, and he
has never since been similarly affected. This was
an extreme case. But do not examples of the want
of sleep, proving very similar results, though in a
very much less degree, occur under our observation
constantly? How altered is the state of mind in
any one of us after even two sleepless nights! Many
a person who under ordinary circumstances is cheerful and unsuspicious, becomes not only irritable and
peevish, but also labors under actual, though tran-
sitory, illusions; such, for example, as thinking that
others neglect him or affront him who have not the
smallest intention of doing either the one or the
other."

Cases similar to the following, which is one of
the passive variety of wakefulness, are by no means
uncommon.

CASE IV.—A lady, aged about thirty-five, unmarried, and of rather delicate constitution, consulted me in regard to persistent wakefulness, with
which she had been affected for nearly a month.
According to the account which she gave me, she
had received a severe mental shock, which had not
lost its influence when a subject of great anxiety
was forced upon her consideration. Her menstrual
period, which had been due about ten days before

she came under my notice, had been anticipated by a week, and the flow was prolonged much above the ordinary time. She had, therefore, lost a good deal of blood, and was, in consequence, greatly reduced in strength. This, conjoined with the exhaustion due to the long-continued wakefulness, rendered her condition a much more serious one than would otherwise have been the case.

She had taken large doses of laudanum, of ether, and of valerian, together with many other medicines, the names of which I do not now recollect, besides employing a variety of means of traditional efficacy. All had, however, been useless. Homœopathy was then tried with an equal want of success. When I first saw her she was nervous and irritable, her hands trembled violently upon the slightest exertion of their muscles, her eyes were bloodshot, the pupils contracted, and the lids opened to the widest possible extent. There was a constant buzzing in the ears, and the sense of hearing was much more acute than was natural. There was also increased sensibility of all that portion of the surface of the body (the skin of the hands, arms, legs, back, and breast) which I submitted to examination with the æsthesiometer. Her pulse was 98, irritable, small, and weak.

At night all her symptoms were increased in violence. Her mind was filled with the most grotesque images which it was possible for the imagination to conceive, and with trains of ideas of the most exaggerated and improbable character. These succeeded each other with a regularity so well marked that she was able to foresee the routine night after night. "No one," she said, "can imagine the weariness I feel, or the horror with which I look forward to the long rows of too familiar phantoms and thoughts which I know will visit me before morning. There is one set," she continued, "which always comes as the clock strikes two. No matter what may be passing through my mind it is banished by this. It consists of a woman with very long hair, who sits on a rock by the sea-side, with her face buried in her hands. Presently a man armed with a long sword comes up behind her, and, clutching her by the hair, drags her to the ground. He puts his knee on her breast, and still holding her hair, cuts it off, and binds her with it, hand and foot. He then commences to pile stones on her, and continues to do so till she is entirely covered, notwithstanding her piercing shrieks, which I hear as distinctly as I do real sounds. Turning then to the sea he cries out, 'Julia, you are avenged. My vow is accomplished. Come! come!' He then draws a dagger from his breast and stabs himself to the heart. He falls over the pile of stones he has raised, and instantly hundreds of little devils not more than a foot high swarm around his body, and finally carry it off through the air. My horror at all this is extreme. For more than an hour the scene is passing before me, and though I know it is all purely imaginary, I cannot shake off the terror it induces."

I questioned this lady closely, and found that she was very intelligent, and fully sensible of the unreality of all her visions. There was no evidence whatever of the slightest tendency to insanity, but there was a condition present which would surely terminate in the loss of her reason if not quickly removed. I regarded her symptoms as indicating a state of passive cerebral congestion, and as calling for stimulants rather than what are called sedatives. I directed, therefore, that she should take an ounce of whisky, properly diluted, every hour, commencing six hours before bedtime; that she should immerse her whole body except her head in water, at the temperature of 98° F., for half an hour just before retiring for the night, and, instead of lying down, should sit up in an easy chair and try to sleep in that position.

I administered the whisky upon the same principle that governs us when we apply stimulating lotions to an inflamed eye, or give alcoholic liquors in passive congestions of other parts of the body. The warm bath was prescribed with a view to its dilating action upon the blood-vessels exposed to its influence; and the sitting position with the object of facilitating the flow of blood from the head, and impeding its return through the carotids and vertebrals.

All these measures I had employed previously with success, in many cases of inability to sleep due to delirium tremens, and which is almost always of the passive or asthenic form. In the instance under consideration their action was all that could be desired. At ten o'clock, having taken the whisky and bath as directed, she sat down to sleep in a comfortable chair, and, as her mother informed me, was asleep in less than half an hour. She awoke about three o'clock, but soon fell asleep again after another dose of whisky, and remained in this condition till about nine o'clock in the morning. She then took breakfast, feeling very much refreshed, but was unable to remain awake longer than two or three hours, but, taking to her chair, slept soundly till evening. That night she was again overcome with sleep, and it was passed very much as was the previous one. No further medicine was required, and after a few nights she went to bed as had been her custom, and slept soundly till morning. Under the use of iron and lager beer she recovered her health and strength.

The foregoing cases are given as examples of the two forms of morbid wakefulness or insomnia to which I wish to call attention. They show that, though the cause in each variety may be essentially the same, the means of relief are not altogether identical. It is important, therefore, to discriminate between them. But the main point upon which it is necessary to insist is, that in morbid wakefulness, whether occurring in strong or weak persons, there is always an excessive amount of blood circulating through the substance of the brain. In the course of the discussion of the points involved in the physiology of sleep, this subject was incidentally noticed. In the following chapter, however, it will be dwelt upon with more particularity.

CHAPTER IX.

THE EXCITING CAUSES OF WAKEFULNESS.

EVERY cause capable of increasing the amount of blood ordinarily circulating through the brain may give rise to wakefulness. As these causes are more or less under the control of the individual, it is important that they should be fully considered.

An increased amount of blood is attracted to the brain, and wakefulness is produced:

1st. *By long-continued or excessive intellectual action, or any powerful emotion of the mind.*—Every organ of the body, the condition of which admits of being ascertained by ocular examination, invariably contains more blood in its tissues when in a state of activity than when its functions are temporarily suspended. We are hence, *a priori,* justified in assuming that the law is equally applicable to the brain, but we are not forced to rely entirely upon reasoning from analogy. It has been shown already that during sleep the circulation of blood within the cranium is at its minimum, both as regards quantity and rapidity, and that as soon as the individual awakes there is an immediate afflux of this fluid to

(240)

the cerebral tissues. All of us are familiar with the facts that, during severe mental labor, or while under the influence of some exciting emotion, the vessels of the head and neck become distended, the head feels full, the face is flushed, and the perspiration of the parts in question is increased in quantity. Within certain limits the more blood there is in the brain the more actively its functions are performed, and so well known is this fact that some persons, who require to exercise the several faculties of the mind to an extreme degree, make use of stimulating ingesta for the purpose of accomplishing the object in view

A moderate degree of cerebral activity is undoubtedly beneficial. Exercise strengthens the mind and improves its faculties, if it is succeeded by a proper period of repose, during which the vessels are emptied to some extent of their contents, and are thus enabled to recover their tone. If, however, the brain is often kept for long periods on the stretch, during which the vessels are filled to repletion, they cannot contract even when the degree of cerebral activity is diminished. Wakefulness results as a necessary consequence, and every day renders the condition of the individual worse, because time also brings the force of habit into operation.

It is not to be denied, however, that many individuals are able to live in comparative health for long periods with but little or no sleep. Thus it is

21

stated* that Boerhaave did not "close his eyes in sleep for a period of *six* weeks, in consequence of his brain being overwrought by intense thought on a profound subject of study." Sir Gilbert Blane† says he was informed by General Pichegru, that for a whole year, while engaged in active campaign operations, he slept but one hour out of the twenty-four. Such statements as these, however, and others to the same effect which have been made, must be accepted with some allowance. Many persons sleep unconsciously, and we all know how common it is for individuals to deny having slept when we have been eye-witnesses of their somnolency. I should consider it impossible for a person to enjoy good health if deprived for even a few weeks of half his ordinary amount of sleep; and it is very probable that Boerhaave's standard of health, never high, was very much lowered by his protracted vigils.

So long as the attention is kept fully aroused, the blood-vessels of the brain are distended, and it is possible for an individual to remain awake while this condition exists. When the attention begins to flag, the tendency is for the vessels to contract, and for sleep to ensue. This disposition may not, however, be strong enough to restore the full meas-

---

* On Obscure Diseases of the Brain, etc. By Forbes Winslow, M.D London, 1860, p. 604.

† Medical Logic, p. 81, quoted in Cyclopedia of Anatomy and Physiology, vol iv. part i. p. 686.

ure of contractility to vessels that have been long overdistended, and then insomnia results.

To this increase in the amount of blood circulating in the brain, many instances of hallucination have been due. It has already been shown that strong mental emotions determine an augmented flow of blood to the cerebral vessels, and cause the production of spectral illusions. In all such cases there is a marked tendency to insomnia present. The account given by Nicolai, a celebrated German bookseller of the last century, of his own disorder, is so interesting and appropriate that I quote it in full. It has never to my knowledge been published in this country.

" During the ten latter months of the year 1790 I had experienced several melancholy incidents which deeply affected me, particularly in September, from which time I suffered an almost uninterrupted series of misfortunes that affected me with the most poignant grief. I was accustomed to be bled twice a year, and this had been done on the 9th of July but was omitted to be repeated at the end of the year 1790. I had, in 1783, been suddenly taken with a violent vertigo, which my physicians attributed to obstructions in the fixed vessels of the abdomen brought on by a sedentary life and a continual exertion of the mind. This indisposition was successfully removed by means of a more strict diet. In the beginning I had found the use of leeches applied to the arms particularly beneficial, and they were afterward repeated two or three times annually when I felt congestions in the head. The last leeches which had been put on previous to the appearance of the phantasms of which I am about to speak, had been applied on the 1st of March, 1790; less blood had consequently been evacuated in 1790 than was usual with me, and from September I was constantly occupied in business which required the most unremitted exertions, and which was rendered still more perplexing by frequent interruptions.

"I had, in January and February of the year 1791, the additional misfortune to experience several extremely unpleasant circumstances, which were followed on the 24th of February by a most violent altercation. My wife and another person came into my apartment in the morning in order to console me, but I was too much agitated by a series of incidents which had most powerfully affected my moral feelings to be capable of attending to them. On a sudden I perceived, at about the distance of ten steps, a form like that of a deceased person. I pointed at it, asking my wife if she did not see it. It was natural that she should not see anything; my question, therefore, alarmed her very much, and she sent immediately for a physician. The phantom continued for about eight minutes. I grew at length more calm, and being extremely exhausted, fell into a restless sleep which lasted about half an hour. The physician ascribed the appearance to violent mental emotion, and hoped there would be no return; but the violent agitation of my mind had in some way disordered my nerves and produced further consequences which deserve a more minute description.

"At four in the afternoon the form which I had seen in the morning reappeared. I was by myself when this happened, and being rather uneasy at the incident, went to my wife's apartment, but there likewise I was accompanied by the apparition, which, however, at intervals disappeared, and always presented itself in a standing posture. About six o'clock there appeared also several walking figures which had no connection with the first.

'After the first day the figure of the deceased person no longer appeared, but its place was supplied by many other phantasms, sometimes representing acquaintances, but mostly strangers. Those whom I knew were composed of living and deceased persons, but the number of the latter was comparatively small. I observed that the persons with whom I daily conversed did not appear as phantasms, these representing chiefly persons who lived at some distance from me.

" These phantasms seemed equally clear and distinct at all times and under all circumstances, both when I was by myself and when I was in company, and as well in the day as at night, and in my own house as well as abroad; they were, however, less frequent when I was in the house of a friend, and rarely appeared to me in the street. When I shut my eyes these phantasms would sometimes vanish entirely, though there were instances when I beheld them with my eyes closed; yet when they disappeared on such occasions, they generally returned when I opened my eyes. I conversed sometimes with my physician and my wife of the phantasms which at the moment surrounded me. They appeared more frequently walking than at rest, nor were they constantly present. They frequently did not come for some time, but always reappeared for a longer or shorter period, either singly or in company, the latter, however, being most frequently the case. I generally saw human forms of both sexes, but they usually seemed not to take the smallest notice of each other, moving as in a market-place where all are eager to pass through the avenue; at times, however, they seemed to be transacting business with each other. I saw also several times people on horseback, dogs and birds. All these phantasms appeared to me in their natural size, and as distinct as if alive, exhibiting different shades of carnation in the uncovered parts as well as different colors and fashions in their dresses, though the colors seemed somewhat paler than in real nature. None of the figures appeared particularly terrible, comical, or disgusting, most of them being of an indifferent shape, and some presenting a pleasing aspect. The longer these phantoms continued to visit me the more frequently did they return, while at the same time they increased in number. About four weeks after they had first appeared, I also began to hear them talk. The phantoms sometimes conversed among themselves, but more frequently addressed their discourse to me: their speeches were commonly short and never of an unpleasant turn. At different times there appeared to me both dear and sensible friends of both sexes, whose addresses tended to appease my grief, which had not yet wholly subsided: their consolatory speeches were in general addressed to me when I was alone. Sometimes, however, I was accosted by these consoling friends while I was engaged in company, and not unfrequently while real persons were speaking to me. These consolatory addresses consisted sometimes of abrupt phrases, and at other times they were regularly executed.

"Though my mind and body were in a tolerable state of sanity all this time, and these phantasms became so familiar to me that they did not cause me the slightest uneasiness, and though I even sometimes amused myself with surveying them, and spoke jocularly of them to my physician and my wife, I yet did not neglect to use proper medicines, especially when they began to haunt me the whole day and even at night, as soon as I waked.

"At last it was agreed that leeches should be again applied to me as formerly, which was actually done, April 20th, 1791, at eleven o'clock in the morning. No person was with me besides the surgeon, but during the operation my chamber was crowded with human phantasms of all descriptions. This continued uninterruptedly till about half an hour after four o'clock, just when my digestion commenced. I then perceived that they began to move more slowly. Soon after their color began to fade, and at seven o'clock they were entirely white. But they moved very little, though the forms were as distinct as before, growing, however, by degrees more obscure yet not fewer in number, as had generally been the case. The phantoms did not withdraw, nor did they vanish, a circumstance which previous to that time, had frequently happened. They now seemed to dissolve in the air, while fragments of some of them continued visible for a considerable time. About eight o'clock the room was entirely cleared of my fantastic visitors.

"Since that time I have felt twice or three times a sensation as if these phantasms were going to reappear, without, however, actually seeing anything. The same sensation surprised me just before I drew up this account, while I was examining some papers relative to these apparitions, which I had drawn up in the year 1791."

While it is doubtless true that variations in the amount of blood in the brain are dependent upon nervous action, it is equally certain that this latter is increased or lessened according as the brain is in a more or less hyperæmic condition. These factors, therefore, react upon each other, and consequently the resulting insomnia is more aggravated than would otherwise be the case.

Instances of insomnia dependent upon intense intellectual exertion have already been given, but the following, which I extract from my note-book, will not, I think, prove uninteresting or uninstructive:

CASE V.—A gentleman, aged thirty-nine, unmarried, of correct habits, and good general health, consulted me on the 19th of April, 1865, in reference to a peculiar nervous affection with which he had suffered for several months. He stated to me that, being engaged upon a literary labor of some importance, he had given the greater part of his time to the studies necessary to its being carried on with success, and was conscious of having overtasked his mental powers. So great, however, was his ambition to excel in his undertaking, that he had persevered notwithstanding the admonitions of friends, and the still more pointed warnings he had received from his own sensations. Instead of sleeping, as had been his custom, from seven to eight hours, he rarely, for nearly a year, had slept more than four hours out of the twenty-four, and frequently even less than this. He did not, however, feel the want of sleep. In fact he was never sleepy, and if this had been the only ill consequence of his severe application I should probably not have had him under my charge at all, so little weight did he attach to the condition which it was of the first importance should be relieved.

The symptom of disordered action which attracted his attention most was an inability to concentrate his mind upon subjects about which he wished to write. There was no difficulty in maintaining a connected line of reasoning, except when he attempted to put his ideas on paper, and then he found it utterly impossible to direct his thoughts in a methodical way. He conversed with me very intelligently in reference to his case, and was perfectly conscious of the difficulty under which he labored. As an instance of the character of his disease, he said that the day before he came to see me he had reflected to his entire satisfaction upon certain points in literature which he was investigating, and that when he came to read over what he had written he found it was a tissue of the most arrant nonsense. The subject of his thoughts was the Greek drama, and the ideas in reference to it, which he communicated to me, were in the highest degree logical and interesting. He then showed me the first page of what he had written, and though he was annoyed at the nonsensical strains of his language, he could not at the same time conceal his amusement at its utter absurdity. I quote a few lines from this paper.

" The rise of the Greek drama is not to be associated with the Homeric age of minstrelsy, nor to be discovered in the Cimmerian darkness of the North. It rests upon a foundation far anterior to either. It is found in the hearts of those men who look beyond a mere utilitarian idea, and who are able to conceive of the existence of beauty without the disturbance due to causes inseparably connected with the barbarism from which Greece emerged into that mythical age which created a god for every river and forest, and for every emotion of the heart or element of the mind. Lyric poetry and philosophy may claim the precedence of antiquity, but the power that could draw tears from eyes that had never before wept, or cause the hardened lines of stoicism to relax in smiles, is not to be despised or even elevated upon a pinnacle of greatness."

At the time of writing, his thoughts flowed so rapidly that he was not conscious of the disconnected nature of his composition. If he stopped, however, to read it over, he at once saw how thoroughly it misrepresented his conceptions. No matter what the subject, the same thing happened, and even the most trivial notes could not be written without language being used which was either perfectly without relation to the ideas he wished to communicate, or else in direct opposition to them. For instance, wishing to obtain a book from a friend, he found he had written the prayer of Socrates which concludes the Phædrus of Plato. On another occasion, intending to indite an epistle to a lady who had sent him a volume of her poems, he discovered, when half through his letter, that he had requested her to accept one of his own books, and had then gone on to give his views relative to suicide and matrimony.

Upon questioning him, I ascertained that he went

to bed generally about two o'clock in the morning; that he lay awake for an hour at least, during which his mind was exceedingly active; and that he rose between six and seven, took a sponge-bath, and ate a light breakfast. He then went to work, spending the day in reading, and in dictating to his sister, who wrote out his language *verbatim*. At six o'clock he dined plainly, and then again resumed his labors. He drank neither tea, coffee, nor any alcoholic liquor. Occasionally he took a cup of chocolate at breakfast.

The only indications of a disordered system other than those I have mentioned were, that his pulse was too frequent (104), that it was irritable and irregular; that he had had several attacks of slight vertigo and headache; that his eyes were brilliant and somewhat congested, and that pressure upon the closed lids caused considerable pain. His bowels, contrary to what might have been reasonably expected, were regular, and his appetite was generally good. His urine contained an excess of urea and of phosphates; oxalate of lime was also present. There was nothing in his condition which appeared to give him the least anxiety, beyond the impossibility of controlling his thoughts when writing, and this he attributed directly to overexertion of his mental powers. He had, however, tried the effect of suspending his studies for two or three weeks, but had not perceived that any benefit was derived from this procedure. He had, therefore, returned to his occupations.

I told him very plainly that, unless he was prepared to forego his literary labors for several weeks at least, he would be in great danger of permanent injury to his mind; but that with the avoidance of severe mental exertion, and by the aid of other measures, I believed he could be restored. He demurred somewhat to the first condition, but finally promised to follow my advice implicitly.

Although I was unable to explain the fact that mental aberration should only be manifested when he wrote, I was confident that his condition was clearly the result of intense hyperæmia of the brain, and that if this could be dissipated, and sound, regular, and sufficient sleep be produced, the mental trouble would also vanish. I therefore directed that half a dozen dry cups should be applied to the nape of the neck every evening, that he should take a warm bath directly afterward, and that, while in the bath, cold water should be poured on his head. Instead of lying down when he attempted to sleep, I advised that he should assume the sitting posture, supporting his head on a hair pillow. All literary labor was to cease. Instead of the books he was in the habit of studying, he was to read novels. He was to compose himself for sleep at eleven o'clock at night, and was to rise punctually at seven; take his sponge-bath as usual, and, after eating a moderate breakfast, to do anything he liked, except studying or writing, till twelve o'clock, when he was to take a walk for an hour, then eat a biscuit,

22

read light literature till four, and then ride on horseback till six, at which hour he was to dine, simply, but to the extent his appetite prompted him. He had been in the habit of smoking one cigar a day (after dinner), and I allowed him to continue in this indulgence.

I am thus particular in stating my instructions, because I determined to see what could be done by hygienic measures, and others directed to the relief of the supposed cerebral congestion, without resorting to the use of drugs, so long as it was probable they would not be required. Opium and other medicines of the narcotic class would, I was satisfied. do more harm than good; bromide of potassium I reserved for use, should it become necessary to employ it.

I have every reason to believe that he complied faithfully with the directions given him, and ere long marks of decided improvement were visible. His pulse had fallen to 80, was regular and full; there was no more headache or vertigo; his eyes had lost their bloodshot appearance, and above all, his sleep had become sound, and was of from seven to eight hours' duration nightly. As soon as he got settled in his easy chair for the night his eyelids began to close, and he slept steadily on till it was time for him to get up for the day. Three weeks were necessary to bring about these results in full, although amendment was manifested from the first. Yesterday, May 18th, I wrote him a note, requesting his permission to make use of his case in illustration of this memoir. The following is his answer: it is the first time he has written a line for a month:

"MY DEAR DOCTOR:—If, in your opinion, my case is possessed of any value in a pathological point of view, I hope you will make such use of it as will best serve the ends of science. I make only one condition. You know I am a literary man, and that my reputation as a student and author would suffer in the estimation of the critics were I suspected of insanity. It takes very little to form a foundation for such an assumption, and, perhaps, in my case, there would be more truth than fiction in the notion as applied to me. With the exception, therefore, of giving my name, you are at perfect liberty to dish me up for the satisfaction of all your medical friends.

"I shall come and see you to-morrow, and in the mean time believe me ever,

"Yours sincerely and gratefully,

"—— —— ——.

"P.S.—I have read the above over, and to my great delight find that I have said what I wanted to say. I would stand on my head with joy, were it not that you were desirous of keeping as much blood out of my noddle as possible. *Laus Deo.* Can I go to work Monday?"

I had no intention of letting him "go to work" on Monday, or for at least two weeks subsequently. I was of the opinion, however, that after that time he could resume his labors to a slight extent, and gradually extend them—not to the limit they formerly reached, but to that degree which, while they would add to his reputation as a man of learning, would not exhaust the organ which it was so essential for his objects to preserve in a condition of unimpaired vigor. The result has been all that either he or myself could have desired.

Case VI.—A youth of fifteen was brought to me by his father, on the 16th of August, to be treated for obstinate wakefulness, the consequence of severe mental exertion at school several weeks previously. He had not attended school since the last of June, but had scarcely slept more than an hour or two each night since that time, according to his own and his father's statement. He was a healthy, well-grown lad, with a good appetite, and nothing unusual in his appearance beyond a slight look of weariness and anxiety in his face. During the day there were no hallucinations of any kind, and toward evening he invariably felt overpowered with sleep. As soon, however, as he lay down he heard voices repeating extracts from the lessons he had recently been learning, and his mind became occupied with imaginary scenes in which the gods and goddesses of mythology and the heroes and poets of antiquity played prominent parts, and the whole power of his attention was thus kept engaged with these and other scenes which were formed with astonishing rapidity. Toward morning he fell into an uneasy slumber, and awoke feeling more weary even than when he had gone to bed.

Medicines, among which opium was the chief, had been employed without success. On the contrary, his condition was manifestly rendered worse through their influence. Laudanum, of which he had taken large quantities, always caused headache, without producing the least amelioration in his symptoms. Notwithstanding the palpable connection which existed between the wakefulness and his former intense mental application, he had been allowed to continue his studies, and when he came to me had a Latin grammar in his hand, which he had been diligently studying in the street railway car!

After some very plain conversation with the father, relative to the great danger to which he was subjecting his son, by thus inordinately taxing his mind, I directed the entire cessation of all studies for the present, and an entire change of associations by a visit to the sea-shore, and free indulgence in bathing, fishing, and other recreations. I likewise advised the use, for a few nights, of small doses of bromide of potassium. My advice was implicitly followed, and a few days since I received a visit from the boy's father, and was told by him that his son's health had been completely restored. I recommended that the visit to the sea-side should be prolonged a week or two, that the return to study should be gradual, and that the boy's eagerness to learn should be somewhat restrained by occupations and amusements requiring but little mental exertion.

CASE VII.—An eminent banker consulted me for the purpose of being, as he said, "put to sleep." He informed me that he was engaged in a series of financial operations which, if successful, would be the means of adding largely to his fortune, but that owing to loss of sleep he was unable to give them that careful and full attention which their importance demanded. "I go to bed," he said, "feeling very much exhausted, and dead with sleep, but I am kept awake nearly the whole night by the activity of my thoughts, which run on with a rapidity which astonishes me. Toward morning I get a little sleep, but I arise unrefreshed, and go to my business with a feeling of fullness in my head, and a sensation of weariness, which altogether unfit me for the duties of the day. The consequence is that I cannot concentrate my attention upon the matters which ought to engage it, and that I am in danger of losing a great deal of money simply from lack of mental power to follow the train of operations which I have set in action."

On examining this gentleman, I found his face flushed, his eyes bloodshot, his pulse small, weak, and frequent (104), and his manner excited. He complained of almost constant vertigo, and a feeling when he walked as though his feet did not rest firmly on the ground or support his entire weight. His appetite was capricious, and he maintained his strength mainly by drinking champagne, of which he imbibed two bottles a day, taking in addition "brandy and soda," as occasion seemed to require.

I informed him that his case was a very simple one, and that I could safely promise to put him to sleep provided he would agree to follow my directions implicitly.

This he said he would do.

I told him that in the first place he must leave town and travel for a week, and in the second place take the oxide of zinc. To the first condition he objected strenuously; but the argument which I adduced, that if he did not he would probably go to an insane asylum within the period specified, somewhat startled him, and he yielded a reluctant consent.

He started off that day, and returned in exactly a week, having, as he said, slept eight hours every night during his absence. All his disagreeable symptoms had disappeared, and he was enabled to resume his business with his mental faculties in their full vigor.

2d. *Those positions of the body which tend to impede the flow of blood from the brain, and at the same time do not obstruct its passage through the arteries, while causing hyperæmia, also produce insomnia.*

Several cases have come under my observation in which the influence of position as affecting the disposition to sleep was well marked. It is very evident that the recumbent posture is more favorable to a state of congestion of the brain than the erect, or semi-erect. Individuals who, by excessive mental exertion, have lessened the contractility of the cerebral vessels, almost always experience great difficulty in getting to sleep after lying down, even though previous to so doing they may have been very drowsy. A gentleman, who was a patient of mine a few weeks since, informed me that several years ago he had an attack of wakefulness, which lasted for three or four months, and which was particularly characterized by inability to sleep while lying in bed. While sitting in his office he would often fall asleep in his chair, and previous to going to bed he would be overcome by drowsiness. The moment, however, that he lay down, his mind was aroused into activity, and all sleepiness disappeared. He left off work, traveled, and in a short time recovered perfectly. It will be recollected that in the other cases I have cited in this memoir, the phenomena were always more strongly marked after the persons affected lay down; and I have always insisted upon the avoidance of the recumbent posture as one of the most important means to be employed in the cure of insomnia. The following is one of the cases referred to above.

CASE VIII.—A gentleman in extensive legal practice requested my advice for persistent wakefulness, with which he had been affected for several weeks, in consequence of unremitting attention to a case in which his sympathies had become greatly interested. For somewhat over a month he had, as he informed me, slept but for an hour or two each day. After dinner he was able to procure this much sleep in his chair, but at night, when he lay down, all his efforts were unavailing. He felt the want of repose very much, and he described the sensation of weariness of body and mind as almost insupportable. So great was this desire for sleep that, notwithstanding repeated disappointments, he was confident each night of being able to secure it, but invariably as soon as he lay down all inclination vanished, and he passed the night in that condition of painful restlessness which had now become horrible to him. There was no very great mental activity, and no hallucinations of sight, but when his head touched the pillow a low buzzing sound, which apparently had its origin in the ears, was heard, and remained there to keep him awake. He could not shut out this noise, no matter how energetically he endeavored to render himself oblivious to it, and all the means, such as opium, chloroform, and alcoholic liquors of various kinds, which he tried in the hope of obtaining relief, only aggravated the difficulty.

His general health, ordinarily excellent, had latterly began to give way. His bowels were torpid, he had little or no appetite, and he was almost daily

subject to severe attacks of headache. He was conscious, too, of a very decided change in his disposition. From having been of rather social tenden-
cies, he had become morose and gloomy, disliking
even the companionship of his most intimate friends.
There was also a very decided impairment of his
memory, and he was sensible of the fact that the
power of concentrating his attention upon subjects
of even minor importance was materially weakened.
In conversation he miscalled names, and misplaced
events and things. Thus he called Pittsburg *Pitts-
town*, said *aunt* several times when he should have
said uncle, and confounded *Newark* with New York.
By attention to hygienic measures, avoidance of the
recumbent position, and the use of moderate doses
of bromide of potassium, he soon obtained a due
amount of sleep, and the other symptoms of a disordered mental and physical organism gradually disappeared.

Dr. Handfield Jones* relates a case in which the
influence of position was strongly marked "A
gentleman aged twenty-four, after considerable
mental strain, experienced the following symptoms·
He was thoroughly weary and drowsy at the close
of the day, and felt, as well he might, the need of
nature's restorer; scarcely, however, had he laid
down his head, when the cerebral arteries began to

---

* Clinical Observations on Functional Nervous Disorders. London, 1864, p. 284.

throb forcibly, and soon all inclination for sleep was banished, and for hours he lay wide awake, but deadly weary.   The *causa mali* here was evidently deficient tonicity in the cerebral arteries, or more exactly paresis of their vasa motor nerves.   As the arteries relaxed they admitted an undue flow of blood to the brain, which goaded the weary tissue to abnormal action."

De Boismont* refers to a case, on the authority of M. Moreau, in which an individual was able to obtain hallucinations of sight by inclining his head a little forward.   By this movement the return of blood from the head was impeded, and thus there was an exaltation of certain of the cerebral functions.   Wakefulness is nothing more than an exaggeration of the normal functions of the brain.   For this organ to act with vigor, an increased flow of blood is necessary.   If this flow is continued, without proper periods of repose, a state of erethism and insomnia is produced.   Instances have been recorded in which persons have found it necessary to assume the recumbent position whenever they had any severe mental labor to perform.   The following extract, bearing upon this point, from a work† already quoted, is interesting:

---

* A History of Dreams, Visions, Apparitions, etc.   American edition.   Philadelphia, 1855.

† The Philosophy of Mystery.   By Walter Cooper Dendy.   London, 1841, page 290.

"The posture of supination will unavoidably induce that increased flow of blood to the brain which, under certain states of this fluid, is so essential to the production of brilliant waking thoughts; and are indeed attained so often by another mode—the swallowing of opium.

"A gentleman of high attainment was constantly haunted by a specter when he retired to rest, which seemed to attempt his life. When he raised himself in bed *the phantom vanished, but reappeared* as he resumed the recumbent position.

"Some persons always retire to bed when they wish to think; and it is well known that Pope was often wont to ring for pens, ink, and paper in the night, at Lord Bolingbroke's, that he might record, ere it was lost, that most sublime or fanciful poesy which flashed through his mind as he lay in bed. Such, also, was the propensity of Margaret, Duchess of Newcastle, who (according to Cibber, or rather Shiel, the *real* author of the 'Lives of the Poets') kept a great many young ladies about her person, who occasionally wrote what she dictated. Some of them slept in a room contiguous to that in which her grace lay, and were ready, at the call of her bell, to rise any hour of the night to write down her conceptions, lest they should escape her memory.

"Henricus ab Heeres (in his 'Obs. Med.') says that when he was a professor he used to rise in the night, open his desk, compose much, shut his desk, and again to bed. On his waking, he was con-

scious of nothing but the happy result of his composition.

"The engineer Brindley even retired to bed for a
day or two, when he was reflecting on a grand or
scientific project.

"I deny not that the darkness or stillness of night
may have had some influence during this inspiration. I may also allow that some individuals compose best while they are walking, but this *peripatetic*
exertion is calculated itself to produce what we term
determination of blood to the head. I have heard of
a most remarkable instance of the power of position
in influencing mental energy in a German student
who was accustomed to study and compose with his
head on the ground, and his feet elevated and resting
against the wall.

"And this is a fragment of a passage from Tissot,
on the subject of monomania.

"——— 'Nous avons vu étudier dans cette acadé-
mie, il n'y a pas long temps, un jeune homme de
mérite, qui *s'étant mis dans la tête* de découvrir la
quadrature du cercle, est mort, fou, à l'Hôtel Dieu
à Paris.'*

---

* It is perhaps scarcely necessary to call attention to the fact that
Mr. Dendy has altogether mistaken the signification of the words in
the above quotation from Tissot, printed in italics. He appears to
think they mean *being put on his head,* a translation which would
make very great nonsense out of the whole extract. The words will
be found in Tissot's *Avis aux Gens de Lettres et aux Personnes séden-
taires sur leur Santé*, Paris, 1768, p. 28, and in English, in a trans-

"You will smile when I tell you that the tints of the landscape are brighter to our eyes if we *reverse the position of the head.*"

Tissot, in the work to which reference has just been made, cites an instance in which position was taken advantage of to solve a problem in mathematics. A gentleman, remarkable for his accuracy in calculation, for a wager *lay down on a bed* and wrought, by mere strength of memory, a question in geometrical progression, while another person, in another apartment, performed the same operation with pen and ink. When both had finished, the one who had worked mentally repeated his product, which amounted to sixteen figures, and, insisting that the other gentleman was wrong, desired him to read over his different products. On this being done he pointed out the place where the first mistake lay, and which had run through the whole. He paid very dearly, however, for gaining his wager, as for a considerable time he had a swimming in his head, pains in his eyes, and severe headaches upon attempting any mathematical labor.

Sir Walter Scott has said somewhere, that the half hour *passed in bed*, after waking in the morning, was the part of the day during which he conceived his best thoughts.

---

lation entitled "*A Treatise on the Diseases of Literary and Sedentary Persons,*" Edinburgh, 1772, p. 26. The work is well worthy of attention even at this day, as containing many most interesting facts and important suggestions.

Dr. Forbes Winslow* makes some excellent remarks upon the relations existing between position and wakefulness. He says:

"In some types of insanity the patient's mind is altogether absorbed in the contemplation of a frightful spectral illusion. Under these circumstances the unhappy sufferer is afraid to close his eyes in sleep from an intense fear and dread that he will then fall an easy prey to the horrible phantasms which his morbid imagination has called into existence, and which, he imagines, follow him in all his movements. The patient so afflicted declares he will not sleep, and resolutely repudiates and perseveringly ignores all disposition to slumber. On many occasions he obstinately refuses to go to bed, or to place himself in a recumbent position. He will battle with his attendant if he attempts to convey him to bed. He insists on remaining in the chair, in standing in an erect position all night, and often determinately walks about the room when those near him are in profound repose. In these cases the hallucinations appear to be most exquisitely and acutely vivid when the patient is placed in a recumbent position, on account, it is supposed, of the mechanical facilities thus afforded for the blood gravitating freely to the head.

"A gentleman who appeared free during the day from any acute hallucinations, never could lie on

* On Obscure Diseases of the Brain, etc., p. 607.

his back without being distressingly harassed by a number of frightful imps, whom he imagined to be dancing fantastically around him during the night. Under these circumstances, undisturbed sleep, while in bed, could never be obtained. He was in the habit of sleeping in an arm-chair for some time in consequence of these symptoms. He, however, eventually recovered, and has been for several years entirely free from all hallucinations."

It has frequently occurred to me to notice the increase in the number and intensity of the hallucinations of patients affected with delirium tremens as soon as they assumed the recumbent position. The difficulty of sleeping is in such cases always correspondingly augmented.

3d. *An increased amount of blood is determined to the brain, and wakefulness is produced by certain substances used as food or medicine.*

Daily experience assures us of the truth of this proposition. In general terms, it may be said that all those substances which, when ingested into the system, increase the force and frequency of the heart's action, cause also a hyperæmic condition of the brain and tend to the supervention of wakefulness.

Chief among these agents are to be placed alcohol, opium, belladonna, stramonium, Indian hemp, tea, and coffee. It is true that the first two of these, when taken in large quantities, sometimes give rise to a comatose condition. This, however, as has already been shown, is not a consequence of an increased amount of blood in the brain, but results from the circulation in that organ of blood which has not been duly oxygenated by respiration. My experiments on this head have been many, and show conclusively that neither alcohol nor opium possesses any stupefying effect, if means be taken to insure the full aeration of the blood. If, however, these substances be administered beyond a certain limit, they so act upon the nerves which supply the respiratory muscles as to interfere with the process of respiration, and hence the blood is not sufficiently subjected to the action of the atmosphere. Unaerated blood therefore circulates in the brain, and coma—not sleep—is produced.

No substance is capable of acting as a direct hypnotic, except that which lessens the amount of blood in the brain. In small doses alcohol and opium do this indirectly, through their stimulating properties exerted upon overdistended blood-vessels, as has been shown in regard to the first named in a case already cited; but they never so act upon the healthy brain. In the normal state of this organ their action in small doses is always that of excitants. The word " small " is of course used in a relative sense. What is a small dose for one person may be a large one for another, and *vice versa*.

In this connection it is scarcely necessary to dwell at any length upon the wakefulness produced by delirium tremens from the excessive ingestion of alcohol or opium. In the *post-mortem* examinations —four only—which I have made of individuals dying from this affection as the result of the immediate use of alcohol, the brain was invariably found congested. Either hyperæmia or its consequence, effusion of serum, is the ordinary pathological condition discovered in such cases.

In regard to opium, most practitioners have doubtless noticed the effect which it and its preparations frequently produce in preventing sleep. I have known one dose of half a grain of opium keep a patient awake for three consecutive days and nights, during the whole of which period intense mental excitement was present. As is well known, the Malays, when they wish *to run amuck*, bring on the necessary degree of cerebral stimulation by the use of opium. During the condition thus produced insomnia is always present. It is certainly true, however, that in moderately large doses opium acts as a direct hypnotic, and the same may be said of other narcotics.

Belladonna, stramonium, and Indian hemp likewise produce congestion of the brain and wakefulness. The latter, under the name of *hashish*,* is

---

* The word *assassin* is derived from the word *hashish*, from the fact that a sect in the East called *Assassins* made use of *hashish* to induce the temporary insanity during which their crimes were perpetrated. See *History of the Assassins*, by the Chevalier Joseph von Hammer, translated from the German by O. C. Wood, M.D., London, 1835, p. 233, note.

still used in the East to bring on a state of delirium, and, if rumor is to be credited, has its votaries in this country. Tea and coffee act in a similar but far less powerful manner. As one of the results of experiments with these substances, instituted upon myself, I found that the circulation of the blood was rendered more active.* Their influence in preventing sleep is well known to the generality of people, and this effect is doubtless entirely due to their action upon the heart and blood-vessels by which the amount of blood in the brain is increased. In persons of fair and thin skins, who are not accustomed to the use of either of these beverages, the face can be seen to flush after they have been taken; and I have frequently met with persons in whom their use was always followed by suffusion of the eyes, and a feeling of fullness within the head. Their power to increase the force and brilliancy of our thoughts, and to sustain the mind under depressing influences, has long been recognized, and is to be ascribed to the same cause as that which prevents sleep.

4th. *Wakefulness is also caused by functional derangements of certain organs of the body, whereby an increase in the amount of blood in the brain is produced.*

Under this head are embraced those cases of sleeplessness due to exalted sensibility of the nervous system. They are chiefly met with in persons of

---

* Physiological Memoirs, 1863, p. 24, *et seq.*

feeble constitution. The slightest impression made upon the skin, or any other organ of sense, is converted into a sensation out of all proportion to the exciting cause. There is thus a condition of general hyperæsthesia which greatly tends to the prevention of sound and refreshing sleep. The following case illustrates very well the phenomena of the state in question:

CASE IX.—A lady recently came under my care for extreme wakefulness, the result, as she correctly supposed, of debility. During the month of August she had resided in a malarious region, and had had a series of attacks of intermittent fever before she would consent to take quinine for its cure. By the time the disease was conquered she had become very much reduced, and her constitution had received a shock from which it will probably not recover for several years. I saw her for the first time on the 26th of September, and she was then so feeble that she was unable to be out of her bed for more than an hour or two each day. Her nervous system was in an exceedingly irritable condition, the least noise startled her, she was unable to bear the full light of day, and so sensitive was her skin, that the light clothes she wore caused her the greatest uneasiness. She informed me that she had scarcely slept for seventeen days and nights, and though I received this statement with some grains of allowance, I was very sure, from her general appearance, that she was suffering from insomnia. At night the feeling of general discomfort was greatly increased, the weight of the bedclothes was insupportable, and she passed the hours tossing restlessly on her bed or in walking the floor. By morning she was feverish, irritable, and thoroughly exhausted. A cup of coffee and a little buttered toast constituted her breakfast, after which she felt somewhat revived.

Conceiving that all the symptoms were referable to debility and passive cerebral congestion, I advised nutritious food, tonics, stimulants, exercise in the open air, the warm bath, cold water to the head, and the avoidance of the recumbent posture. Amendment began almost immediately, and by the end of a week the hyperæsthesia had disappeared, and she slept soundly and sufficiently.

In reference to this form of wakefulness, Dr. Handfield Jones* makes some judicious observations. He says: "A girl recently under my care with very various and marked signs of prostration of nerve-power, suffered for many months with exceedingly restless nights, the cause of which appeared to be chiefly great hyperæsthesia. Although she improved materially in other respects, she did not sleep well until she was removed from London to a healthy part of the country. I have had several patients, two especially, both temperate males, who for a length of time were quite dependent for

---

* On Functional Nervous Disorders. London, 1864, p. 282.

good rest at night on wine taken either on going to bed or in the course of the night. * * * It is not easy to form a precise idea of the state of the nervous centers in which a 'nightcap,' as above mentioned, is so effectual in procuring sleep. Debility is certainly one marked pattern of it, but there must be surely another, even more important, as the most profound debility does not, by any means, always interfere with sound sleep, nay, rather seems to conditionate it. This other element, we are much disposed to think, is hyperæsthesia, or irritability, which, as already noticed, commonly increases *pari passu* with weakness. The condition may be compared with that of neuralgia, when it is beginning to give way under treatment, and is so readily reproduced by anything which causes exhaustion. Now, as the stimulant recruits the exhansted nerve-force, the hyperæsthesia ceases, and the brain tissue subsides into a state of calm repose. It may be added here that it is often well to give not only a stimulant, but also some digestible nourishment about the time of going to rest, or even in the course of the night when debility to a serious extent exists. It is quite certain that a craving empty stomach is by no means favorable to quiet slumber, and in this point of view moderate suppers are far from being unsuitable to many invalids. I well remember the case of a lady who, the night after a natural confinement, woke up with severe gastric disorder and flatulence, which resisted various medications, but subsided immediately after a plate of cold meat and some brandy and water. Among the various soporifics, I doubt if there be any more potent, especially for the weakly and hyperæsthetic, than prolonged exposure to the cold open air. This should be so managed as not to cause great fatigue, and if well timed and followed by a sufficient meal, it will be found an admirable preparation for sound nightly slumber."

In the foregoing remarks it is perceived that Dr. Jones fails to recognize the state of passive congestion of the brain which in cases such as he describes, and in many similar ones which have come under my care, is almost invariably present. It is this feature which, in addition to the debility, gives so marked a character to the species of insomnia under consideration. The hyperæsthesia, like the wakefulness, is merely a result of the cerebral hyperæmia.

Several cases of insomnia, the result of disordered menstruation, have come under my observation. We can very well understand how, in women suffering from suppression of this function, a slight degree of cerebral hyperæmia and consequent wakefulness should result. About the climacteric time of life, when irregularities in the menstrual flow are very common, there is quite generally extreme sleeplessness as each period approaches, which is not ordinarily relieved till the catamenia make their appearance. In such cases measures directed to the relief of the existent congestion of the brain will generally prove effectual in causing natural sleep.

Irregular or deficient action of the heart and blood-vessels is a frequent cause of wakefulness. One of the principal results of such disordered action of the circulatory organs is coldness of the extremities, and an attendant condition of repletion of the central vessels. As a consequence there is in these cases almost invariably great wakefulness. As Dr. Cheyne* has remarked, many a delicate female, from going to bed with cold feet, is deprived of hours of sleep in the early part of the night, and thereby falls into nervous complaints, obstinate dyspepsia, and uterine irregularity, who might have escaped had the circulation of the surface of the body been properly sustained.

There are cases, however, of habitual cold feet, accompanied by wakefulness, which are not so much due to deficient power in the heart as to disordered nervous action. But, whatever the cause, there is always, while the condition exists, an excessive amount of blood in the cranial vessels. An instance of the kind came under my observation several years ago in the person of an army officer, of strong constitution and otherwise of good health. Heat applied to the extremities gave only temporary relief, and stimulants taken internally were equally inefficacious. He was finally entirely cured by the

---

* Cyclopedia of Practical Medicine, vol. iv., art. Wakefulness.

repeated passage of the direct galvanic current through the sciatic and crural nerves and their branches.

Indigestion is quite a common cause of wakeful ness, even when no marked disagreeable sensations are experienced in the digestive organs. A full meal, especially if it be of highly seasoned or otherwise improper food, will often keep the offending individual awake the greater part of the night. We know that apoplexy is especially apt to occur soon after the stomach has been overloaded with food. The return of the blood from the head is impeded, and the rupture of an intercranial vessel, or an effusion of serum, is the result of the cerebral congestion. Insomnia is a milder effect of the same cause.

There are several other abnormal conditions of the system in which wakefulness plays an important part, but their consideration would lead us into the discussion of the phenomena of many diseases of which it is simply a symptom, or of secondary consequence. The remarks which have been made in regard to it have reference to its existence as an evidence of slight cerebral congestion, and therefore as being of sufficient importance to demand the aid of both physician and patient in effecting its cure.

CHAPTER X.

THE principles which should prevail in the treatment of wakefulness are indicated to some extent by the remarks which have already been made. It the views which I have given relative to the pathology of this affection be correct, there can be no doubt in regard to the means to be employed for its cure. Happily, theory and practice are in perfect accord in respect to the therapeutical measures to be adopted. These may be arranged into two classes:

1st. Those which by their tendency to soothe the nervous system, or to distract the attention, diminish the action of the heart and blood-vessels, or correct irregularities in their function, and thus lessen the amount of blood in the brain.

2d. Those which directly, either mechanically or through a specific effect upon the circulatory organs, produce a similar effect.

Under the first head are embraced many agencies which from time immemorial have been known to cause sleep. Among them are music, monotonous sounds, gentle frictions of the surface of the body, soft undulatory movements, the repetition by the

(278)

insomnolent of a series of words till the attention is diverted from the exciting emotion which engages it, and many others of similar character which individuals have devised for themselves. In slight cases the measures belonging to this class often prove effectual, but in persistent insomnia they are generally altogether nugatory.

Under the second head we shall find comprehended the means which are chiefly to be relied on in the treatment of cases of morbid wakefulness.

Chief among them are embraced those measures which tend to improve the general health of the patient, and which are chiefly of a hygienic character. Whatever causes produce an irritable condition of the nervous system, indirectly at least increase the disposition to wakefulness. It is important, therefore, that these should be thoroughly understood and avoided, and I accordingly propose to consider them at some length.

Food.—While it is an error to suppose, as is generally done, that a moderately full meal, eaten shortly before bedtime, is necessarily productive of wakefulness, there is no doubt that this condition is induced by an excessive quantity of irritating or indigestible food. A hearty supper of plainly cooked and nutritious food rather predisposes to sleep. Most of us have experienced the drowsiness which so often follows dinner. This is due to the fact that the process of digestion requires an increased amount of blood in the organs which perform it, and consequently the brain receives a less quantity. A tendency to sleep is therefore induced. It is a natural and healthy predisposition, and when yielded to moderately conduces to a more complete assimilation of the food than would otherwise take place. When, however, the food ingested is not such as is merely sufficient for the wants of the system, but is inordinate in amount, or irritating in quality, the hypnotic effect is neutralized, and often a state of wakefulness supervenes, from the fact that the quantity of blood circulating in the brain is augmented instead of being diminished. This last result is induced either by the pressure of the overloaded stomach upon the abdominal vessels or through a reflex action on the heart, by which it is excited to increased activity.

In young children, who are very susceptible to the influence of causes acting upon the nervous system, we often see both sleep and wakefulnesss result as direct effects of eating. When the quantity of milk taken has not been excessive, the child quietly drops asleep at the breast. On the contrary, when a superabundance has been ingested, it either remains awake or the sleep is disturbed. In adults it is, as has already been mentioned, not uncommon for apoplexy to ensue upon a large meal of improper food.

In order, therefore, that a disposition to wakefulness may be removed, it is essential that attention should be paid to the diet of the affected individual.

As a rule, people are underfed. This is especially the case with women, who too generally indulge in what may be called "slops," to the exclusion of good, solid, nutritious food derived in great part from the animal kingdom. By such a faulty diet the tone of the system is lowered, and local congestions of different parts of the body are produced. If the brain be one of these, wakefulness results.

Most of the cases of insomnia which occur in women are of the passive variety, and require not only nutritious food, but *stimulants* Of the latter, *whisky* is generally to be preferred as acting rapidly, as less likely to disagree with the stomach than many kinds of wine, and as being purer than the stuff ordinarily sold as brandy. As a good stimulant, and at the same time tonic, nothing can be preferable to *Tarragona wine*, drunk at dinner to the extent of a glass or two. It possesses all the essential qualities of pure port, and is much more reli-, able and wholesome than the mixture of elderberry juice and alcohol which passes for this latter wine. Next to Tarragona wine must be ranked good *lager beer.*

Although the effect of *coffee* is generally such as to induce sleeplessness, there are cases in which its action is directly the reverse. I have had several slight cases of passive wakefulness under my care which were entirely and speedily cured by a cup of strong coffee taken for three or four nights in succession at bedtime. It is especially useful in females

24*

of languid circulation, and a consequent tendency to internal congestions.

Stimulants such as those mentioned, and others which might be noticed, it must be clearly understood are only useful in the asthenic or passive form of insomnia; in the sthenic or active form of the affection they are altogether inadmissible, and if employed will certainly increase the difficulty.

The good effects of moderate but regular *physical exercise* in dissipating wakefulness can scarcely be overestimated. It is almost impossible to produce any permanently beneficial influence without the aid of this powerful tonic. To be of any material service, the exercise should be taken in the open air and should extend to the point of inducing a slight feeling of fatigue.

The *warm bath* is also a very valuable means of determining blood from the head, and calming nervous irritability. Frequently, especially in children, I have found that simply putting the feet in water of the temperature of 100° F. has been sufficient to induce a sound and healthy sleep, when laudanum and other means have failed.

Cold water, applied directly to the scalp, is often of great effect in diminishing the amount of blood in the brain. It is not admissible in the asthenic form of wakefulness. When the individual is strong, the heart beating with force and frequency, and the mental excitement great, its influence is almost invariably good. The exact temperature is a matter for the judgment of the physician. I have often used it as cold as ice could make it, 32° F., or thereabouts.

In the action of cold water, applied to the head in cases of insomnia, we have another proof of the real nature of this affection. It is known that in Thibet mothers place their wakeful children in such positions as will admit of a small stream of cold water falling from a slight elevation upon the head. I have in some work—on which I cannot now lay my hands—read a very full account of this custom, and seen a cut representing the process. The children very soon fall into a quiet sleep. I have often seen the application of the cold *douche* to the heads of refractory prisoners bring on a deep sleep.

The effects of *position* in aid of other remedies have also been alluded to. I make use of its advantages in all severe cases of insomnia which come under my charge, and we have, in its efficacy, additional confirmation of the correctness of the theory that the condition of the brain in such cases is one of hyperæmia.

Among the more purely medicinal agents, *bromide of potassium* occupies the first place, and can almost always be used with advantage to diminish the amount of blood in the brain, and to allay any excitement of the nervous system that may be present in the sthenic form of insomnia. That the first named of these effects follows its use, I have recently ascertained by experiments upon living animals, the details of which will be given at another time. Suffice it now to say, that I have administered it to dogs whose brains had been exposed to view by trephining the skull, and that I have invariably found it to lessen the quantity of blood circulating within the cranium, and to produce a shrinking of the brain from this cause. Moreover, we have only to observe its effects upon the human subject to be convinced that this is one of the most important results of its employment. The flushed face, the throbbing of the carotids and temporals, the suffusion of the eyes, the feeling of fullness in the head, all disappear as if by magic under its use. It may be given in doses of from ten to thirty grains—the latter quantity is seldom required, but may be taken with perfect safety in severe cases.

Another very admirable preparation is the *oxide of zinc*. This substance appears to be especially beneficial in those cases of wakefulness due to excessive mental exertion or anxiety of mind. I usually prescribe it in doses of two grains, three times a day, the last dose being taken just at bedtime.

Opium I very seldom employ in the treatment of wakefulness, from the facts that its effects vary so greatly in accordance with the dose, and that its action is not limited to the simple induction of sleep. There are cases, however, in which its influence is decidedly beneficial. Care should be taken to give it in sufficiently large but not excessive quantities.

The influence of opium in lessening the amount of blood in the brain is very distinctly recognized by Dr. Handfield Jones, and also by Dr. Alfred Stillé.* Both these authors account in this manner for its hypnotic effect. As has been shown, my own experiments tend strongly to confirm this reasoning.

Hyoscyamus is more generally admissible. It is especially indicated in those cases which are accompanied by great nervous irritability. It is difficult to obtain any preparation of this drug which retains its virtues. I have usually employed the tincture in doses of from one to two drachms. I do not think, however, that it possesses any advantages over bromide of potassium, or that it is even equal in any respect to this agent.

In regard to *valerian, assafœtida*, and other *antispasmodics*, I have nothing to say in commendation. *Tonics* are, however, almost always useful, even in the active form of the affection. Among them *quinine* and *iron* are more generally indicated.

When wakefulness is a consequence of functional derangement of distant organs, the measures of relief must be directed to the cure of the primary disease, in order to produce any permanent alleviation of the cerebral difficulty.

In those cases of insomnia dependent upon severe and long-continued mental exertion, all means will

* Therapeutics and Materia Medica, 2d edition, Philadelphia, 1864, vol. ii. page 659.

fail to remedy the trouble unless the affected individual consents to use his brain in a rational manner. Proper intervals of relaxation should be insisted upon, and in some cases it may be necessary to suspend all intense intellectual effort for a time. When the means will permit, travel can always be undertaken with advantage. It is surprising sometimes to see how rapidly the brain recovers its tone, and the system generally recuperates through the change of associations and scenes incident to travel.

The disposition of the age seems to be to ignore the fact that the nervous system can exhaust itself by excessive intellectual labor. A short time since intelligence was received from abroad that one of the most distinguished men of Great Britain had committed suicide, in consequence of insanity produced by overexertion of his mind. Thus one more victim is added to the long list of those who have disregarded the laws of their being; and again we are reminded that there is a limit to the exercise of our intellectual powers, beyond which we cannot pass with safety.*

---

* The instance alluded to, that of Admiral Fitzroy, is thus commented upon by the *Spectator* of May 6th, 1865:

"Admiral Fitzroy, the well-known meteorologist, committed suicide on Monday morning at his own house. He had overworked himself of late; found that he was losing his memory; became sleepless, and resorted to opium to obtain ease, which aggravated his symptoms. His doctor had warned him that he ran great risk of paralysis, but from a false tenderness did not at once compel him to give up labor."

The *London Review* of the same date says: "He (Admiral Fitzroy) acquired that terrible inability to sleep, which is one of the most dreadful of those means by which nature avenges the abuse of the mental powers, and he was forced to take opium at night; at one time to an extent which threatened serious consequences."

CHAPTER XI.

SOMNOLENCE.

SOMNOLENCE or drowsiness is generally regarded, when persistent, as being more strongly indicative of organic changes in the structure of the brain than is any other derangement of sleep.

This opinion is mainly, if not entirely, due to the fact that it is confounded with stupor, from which, both in its causes and effects, as has already been shown, it differs in every essential respect.

Somnolence is nothing more than an inordinate tendency to sleep. When manifested in a slight degree it is difficult, without careful examination and a thorough inquiry into the history of the case, to distinguish it from moderate stupor. It is of course very important that the distinction should be made; for, in reality, somnolence is ordinarily no very serious disorder, and is generally symptomatic of eccentric disease, whereas stupor almost invariably results from organic brain affections, from cerebral injuries, or the circulation of poisoned blood through the encephalic blood-vessels.

Whatever lessens the amount of blood normally circulating through the cerebral vessels, tends to the production of somnolence. It is hence a condition

(288)

frequently witnessed in those whose powers of life have been reduced by long-continued disease, by excesses of various kinds, or by affections which essentially consist in enfeeblement of the organism. It is generally met with in the aged, in whom the circulatory organs have lost their pristine vigor.

Many cases of very troublesome and persistent somnolence, having an origin such as I have mentioned, have come under my notice: ordinarily they present no difficult features of treatment, the indications being to increase the tone of the system by stimulants, tonics, nutritious food, and moderate exercise in the open air. These measures will invariably succeed if there be no organic difficulty.

Somnolence, however, is sometimes due to structural changes which interfere with the free passage of blood through the cerebral vessels. It may hence be caused by emboli, which, obstructing the arteries, prevent the normal amount of blood reaching the brain substance. It may also be caused by tumors, which, pressing on the arteries supplying the brain, act in like manner. In such cases it is of secondary importance.

A very curious affection, known as the "Sleepy Disease," has been described as endemic in certain regions of Africa. The following extract* gives a graphic description of the malady:

"Having procured a guide, we crossed the river,

---

* Journal of an African Cruiser, quoted in Curiosities of Modern Travel, London, 1846, p. 239.

and at the mouth of Logan's Creek we exchanged our boat for a large canoe, in which we followed the windings of the deep and narrow inlet for nearly two miles. This brought us to a village of six huts. Without ceremony we entered the dwelling of the old queen (who was busied about her household affairs), and looked around for her granddaughter, to see whom was the principal object of our excursion. On my former visit to Maumee's town, four or five months ago, this girl excited a great deal of admiration by her beauty and charming simplicity. She was then thirteen or fourteen years of age—a bright mulatto, with large and soft black eyes, and the most brilliantly white teeth in the world. Her figure, though small, is perfectly symmetrical. She is the darling of the old queen, whose affections exhaust themselves upon her with all the passionate fire of her temperament, and the more unreasonably because the girl's own mother is dead.

"We entered the hut, as I have said, without ceremony, and looked about us for the beautiful granddaughter; but, on beholding the object of our search, a kind of remorse and dread came over us, such as often affects those who intrude upon the awfulness of slumber. The girl lay asleep in the adjoining apartment, on a mat that was spread over the hard ground, and with no pillow beneath her cheek. One arm was by her side, the other above her head, and she slept so quietly, and drew such imperceptible breath, that I scarcely thought her alive.

"With some little difficulty she was aroused, and awoke with a frightened cry,—a strange and broken murmur,—as if she were looking dimly out of her sleep, and knew not whether our figures were real, or only the fantasies of a dream. Her eyes were wild and glassy, and she seemed to be in pain. While awake, there was a nervous twitching about her mouth and in her fingers; but, being again extended upon the mat, and left to herself, these symptoms of disquietude passed away, and she almost immediately sank again into the deep and heavy sleep in which we found her. As her eyes gradually closed their lids, the sunbeams struggling through the small crevices between the reeds of the hut glimmered down about her head. Perhaps it was only the nervous motion of her fingers, but it seemed as if she were trying to catch the golden rays of the sun and make playthings of them, or else to draw them into her soul and illuminate the slumber that looked so misty and dark to us.

"This poor doomed girl had been suffering—no, not suffering; for, except when forcibly aroused, there appeared to be no uneasiness,—but she had been lingering two months in a disease peculiar to Africa: it is called the 'Sleepy Disease,' and is considered incurable. The persons attacked by it are those who take little exercise, and live principally on vegetables, particularly cassady and rice. Some ascribe it altogether to the cassady, which is supposed to be strongly narcotic—not improbably the climate has much influence, the disease being most prevalent in low and marshy situations. Irresistible drowsiness continually weighs down the patient, who can be kept awake only for the few moments necessary to take a little food. When this lethargy has lasted three or four months, death comes with a tread that the patient cannot hear—and makes the slumber but a little more sound.

"I found the aspect of Maumee's beautiful granddaughter inconceivably affecting. It was strange to behold her so quietly involved in sleep from which it might be supposed she would awake so full of youthful life, and yet to know that this was no refreshing slumber, but a spell in which she was fading away from the eyes that loved her. Whatever might chance, be it grief or joy, the effect would be the same. Whoever should shake her by the arm—whether the accents of a friend fell fully on the ear, or those of strangers like ourselves, —the only response would be that troubled cry, as of a spirit that hovered on the confines of both worlds and could have sympathy with neither. And yet, withal, it seemed so easy to cry to her, 'Awake! Enjoy your life! Cast off this noontide slumber!' But only the peal of the last trumpet will summon her out of that mysterious sleep."

Another and later account of this singular disease has recently been given by M. Dumoutier,* surgeon in the French Navy.

* Gazette des Hôpitaux, Oct. 13, 1868.

According to this observer, the affection commonly called the "sleep-disease" (maladie du sommeil) is met with only among the negroes of the
coast, and principally those of the Gaboon and of
Congo, becoming more rare towards the north. The
most prominent symptoms are an irresistible tendency to sleep, and a feeling of torpor and numbness.
The patient does not complain of pain, and yet there
is a general weakness of the limbs, the gait is totter-
ing, the sensibility is perverted, and the hands imper-
fectly grasp the objects they attempt to seize. During
the sleep the fecal matters and the urine are passed
involuntarily. The respiration is normal, and the
digestion regular. These were the principal symptoms observed in those cases which came under M.
Dumoutier's notice : observing the disease only in
the persons of captives coming from the interior, he
ascribes it to nostalgia, *ennui*, and other moral causes.
Two autopsies made by his colleagues revealed no
abnormal condition of the brain, the spinal cord, or
their membranes.

The treatment employed—quinia, strychnia, and
iron—had no effect. A temporary improvement was
obtained by causing the patients to take part in
the amusements of their companions. Electricity
seemed likewise to retard somewhat the progress of
the disease.

The fact that no organic difficulty of the brain
was discovered after death, is strong proof that the
somnolency was due to some cause affecting the in-

tra-cranial circulation. That the amount of blood was lessened, and that thus a permanent anæmia of the brain was produced, can scarcely be doubted, when regard is had to the observations and experiments recorded in the foregoing pages of this work. Probably the primary derangement was seated in the sympathetic nerve and its ganglia, it having been well settled by familiar observations, and by recent contributions to physiology and pathology, that one of the chief functions of this system is to regulate the caliber of the blood-vessels, and thus to determine the amount of blood circulating through an organ or part of the body.

Numerous cases of protracted sleep are on record. Some of them are evidently fanciful and exaggerated but others are doubtless well founded. One of the most remarkable of these is related, among many others, by Wanley.*

"One Samuel Chelton, of Finsbury, near Bath, a laboring man, about twenty-five years of age, of a robust habit of body, not fat, but fleshy, and of dark-brown hair, happened, on the 13th of May, 1694, and without visible cause, to fall into a very profound sleep, out of which he could by no means be aroused by those about him till after a month's time, when he arose of himself and went to his husbandry business as usual. He slept, ate, and drank as before,

---

* Wonders of the Little World, etc., London, 1806, vol. ii. p. 394; quoted from Universal Magazine, vol. viii. p. 312.

but did not speak a word till about a month after. All the time he slept, victuals and drink stood by him, which were spent every day, and used by him, as was supposed, though no person saw him eat or drink all the while. After this period he continued free from drowsiness or sleepiness till the 9th of April, 1696, when he fell into his sleeping fit again, as he had done before. After some time his friends were prevailed on to try what effect medicines might have upon him. Accordingly, Mr. Gills, an apothecary, bled, blistered, cupped, and scarified him, and used all the external irritating medicines he could think of, but to no purpose; and after the first fortnight he was never observed to open his eyes: victuals stood by him as before, which he ate of now and then, but no one ever saw him eat or evacuate, though he did both very regularly, as he had occasion; and sometimes he was found fast asleep with the pot in his hand in bed, and sometimes with his mouth full of meat. In this manner he lay about ten weeks, and then he could eat nothing at all, for his jaws seemed to be set, and his teeth clinched so close that, notwithstanding all the art that could be used with instruments, his mouth could not be opened to put anything into it to support him. At last, those about him observing a hole in his teeth, made by holding his pipe, they now and then poured some tent into his mouth through a quill. And this was all he took for six weeks and four days; but it amounted to no more than three pints or two quarts.

He had made water only once, and never had a
stool all that time.

"On the 7th of August, which was seventeen weeks
from the 9th of April, when he began to sleep, he
awaked, put on his clothes, and walked about the
room, not knowing he had slept above a night; nor
could he be persuaded he had lain so long, till, going
into the fields, he found everybody busy getting in
their harvest, and he remembered very well when
he fell asleep that they were sowing their barley and
oats, which he then saw ripe and fit to be cut down.
There was one thing remarkable: though his blood
was somewhat wasted with lying so long in bed and
fasting for about six weeks, yet a gentleman assured
Dr. Oliver that when he saw him—which was the
first day of his coming abroad—he looked brisker
than ever he saw him in his life before; and on asking him whether the bed had made him sore, he
assured this gentleman that he never felt this or
any other inconvenience, and that he had not the
least remembrance of anything that passed, or what
was done to him, all that while.   So that he went
again to his husbandry, as he was wont to do, and
remained well till August 17th, 1697, when, in the
morning, he complained of a shivering and a coldness in his back.   He vomited once or twice, and
the same day fell into his sleeping fit again. Dr.
Oliver, going to see him, found him asleep, with a
cup of beer and a piece of bread and cheese upon a
stool by his bed, within his reach.   The doctor felt

his pulse, which at that time was regular, and he also found his heart beat very regular, and his breathing easy and free. The doctor only observed that his pulse beat a little too strong. He was in a breathing sweat, and had an agreeable warmth all over his body. The doctor then put his mouth to his ear, and called him as loud as he could several times by his name, pulled him by the shoulders, pinched his nose, stopped his nose and mouth together as long as he could without choking him, but to no purpose, for all this time he did not give the least sign of being sensible. The doctor lifted up his eyelids, and found his eyeballs drawn up under his eyebrows and fixed without any motion. The doctor then held under one nostril, for a considerable time, a vial with spirits of sal ammoniac, extracted from quicklime; he then injected it several times up the same nostril; and though he had poured into it almost half an ounce of this fiery spirit, it only made his nose run, and his eyelids shiver and tremble a little. The doctor, finding no success with this, crammed that nostril with white powder of hellebore, and waited some time in the room to see what effects all these together might have upon him; but he never gave any sign that he felt what the doctor had done, nor discovered any manner of uneasiness, by stirring any part of his body, that the doctor could observe.

"After all these experiments the doctor left him, being pretty well satisfied that he was asleep, and no sullen counterfeit, as some people supposed. On the doctor's relating what he had observed, several gentlemen from Bath went out to see him, and found him in the same condition the doctor had left him in the day before, only his nose was inflamed and very much swelled, and his lips and the inside of his nostrils were blistered and scabby, occasioned by the spirits and the hellebore. About ten days after the doctor had seen him, Mr. Woolner, an apothecary, finding his pulse beat very high, drew about fourteen ounces of blood from the arm, and tied it up, and left it as he found him; and Mr. Woolner assured the doctor that he never made the least motion when he pricked him, nor all the while his arm was bleeding. Several other experiments were tried by those who went to see him from Bath, but all to no purpose. The doctor saw him again the latter end of September, and found him just in the same position, lying in his bed, but his pulse now was not so strong, nor had he any sweats, as when the doctor saw him before. He tried him again by stopping his nose and mouth, but to no purpose; and a gentleman ran a large pin into his arm to the very bone, but he gave no signs of his being sensible to what was done to him. During all this time the doctor was assured that nobody had seen him either eat or drink, though they watched him as closely as possible,—but food and drink always stood by him, and they observed that sometimes once a day, and sometimes once in two days, all was gone. It was further observed that he never dirtied his bed, but always went to the pot. In this manner he lay till the 19th of November, when his mother, hearing him make a noise, immediately ran up to him and found him eating. She asked him how he did. He replied, 'Very well, thank God.' She asked him again which he liked best, bread and butter, or bread and cheese. He answered, 'Bread and cheese.' Upon .this the woman, overjoyed, left him to acquaint his brother, and both coming straight up into the chamber to speak to him, they found him as fast asleep as ever, and could not by any means awake him. From this time to the end of January, or beginning of February, he did not sleep so profoundly as before; for, when they called him by his name, he seemed to hear them, and became somewhat sensible, though he could not make them any answer. His eyes were not shut so close, and he had frequently great tremblings of his eyelids, upon which they expected every day that he would awake, which did not happen till about the time mentioned, when he awoke perfectly well, but remembered nothing that had happened all the while. It was observed that he was very little· altered in his flesh; he only complained that the cold hindered him more than usual, but he presently went to his labor, as he had done before."

The case of Mary Lyall is quoted by Macnish, from the 8th volume of the Transactions of the Royal Society of Edinburgh, as follows:*

---

* Op. cit.

" This woman fell asleep on the morning of the
27th of June, and continued in that state till the
evening of the 30th of the same month, when she
awoke and remained in her usual way till the 1st of
July, when she again fell asleep, and continued so
till the 8th of August. She was bled, blistered, im-
mersed in the hot and cold bath, and stimulated in
almost every possible way, without having any consciousness of what was going on. For the first
seven days she continued motionless, and exhibited
no inclination to eat. At the end of that time she
began to move her left hand, and, by pointing to her
mouth, signified a wish for food. She took readily
what was given to her. Still she evinced no symptoms of hearing, and made no other kind of bodily
movement than of her left hand. Her right hand
and arm particularly appeared completely dead and
bereft of feeling, and even when pricked with a pin,
so as to draw blood, never shrunk in the least degree. At the same time she instantly drew back
her left arm whenever it was touched by the point
of the pin. She continued to take food whenever it
was offered to her. For the first two weeks her
pulse generally stood at 50, during the third and
fourth week about 60, and on the day before her
recovery at 70 or 72. Her breathing was soft and
almost imperceptible, but during the night-time she
occasionally drew it more strongly, like a person who
has just fallen asleep. She evinced no symptom of
hearing till about four days before her recovery.

On being interrogated after this event upon her extraordinary state, she mentioned that she had no knowledge of anything that had happened—that she had never been conscious of either having needed or received food, or of having been blistered; and expressed most surprise on finding her head shaved. She had merely the idea of having passed a long night in sleep."

Many other cases might be referred to; but as their general features are similar to the two cited, it is unnecessary to quote them. The following instance occurring in this country presents some features of interest. It is reported by Dr. C. A. Hart,[*] of this city.

"Miss Susan C. Godsy, aged 22, of bilious temperament, has been in a somnolent state since 1849, being then eight years of age. Up to within a year of that period she had enjoyed excellent health, she being then attacked with intermittent fever, in the treatment of which opium was extensively used. This was erroneously supposed to have induced her present condition. Soon after her recovery, excessive somnolency began to develop itself, which in 1857 became more profound after an attack of scarlatina anginosa, followed by measles. The lucid intervals will occur from four to six times a day, and last for from five to six minutes; at which periods she will generally take some nourishment, and then

---

[*] New York Medical Journal, December, 1867.

relapse into a profound slumber, from which it is impossible to arouse her.

"In point of general physique there is nothing specially worthy of note, except the comparative plumpness during such a long maintenance of the recumbent posture, with very little muscular exercise. She is about the average height of her sex, with cranial development possibly a little in excess. The hands and feet are both exceedingly small, the nails of which have not grown any since her present condition began.

   *   *   *   *   *   *   *   *

"The catamenia commenced between the fourteenth and fifteenth years, and are generally very irregular and painful ; but, when anything like regularity is attained, the flow occurs about every six weeks.   *   *   *   *   *   *   *

"None of the special senses are in the least diminished or perverted; there has been neither squinting nor excessive dilatation of the pupils. The irides both respond readily to the stimulus of light. While interrogating the mother, a convulsive movement of the entire body took place, apparently more violent in the upper than in the lower extremities. The arms, hands, and feet were in rapid motion. At the subsidence of this, consciousness was established; and the young lady herself, being questioned about her condition, replied in a clear and comprehensible manner, though merely using monosyllables. When asked if she suffered any pain in her head, she replied yes, but without locating it; if in the back, yes; if about the chest or abdomen, no. She was lucid about five minutes, during which time a number of questions were asked her, but without eliciting any further information. She took no food or medicine during this interval of consciousness, and went to sleep while being questioned, remaining in that state during the rest of the time we were there—about half an hour—her rest being perfectly tranquil with the exception of a slight convulsive movement.''

These cases of protracted sleep present many analogies with the condition of hibernation which certain of the lower animals enter into at stated periods. Doubtless the state of the brain is the same, and is one of anæmia.

It has never been my fortune to witness a case of protracted sleep. Regarding the starting-point of the disorder as being situated in the sympathetic system, I should be disposed to employ the direct galvanic current in the treatment—placing the positive pole over the sympathetic nerve in the neck, and the negative over the opposite scapula. This I would do, using a battery of thirty-two or a less number of pairs, every day, for from five to ten minutes.

CHAPTER XII.

SOMNOLENTIA, OR SLEEP DRUNKENNESS.

By somnolentia, or sleep drunkenness, is understood a condition in which some of the mental faculties and senses are fully aroused, others partially so, while others remain as they are in profound sleep. It is therefore an imperfect sleep, or rather a combination of wakefulness and sleep. The phenomena peculiar to it are frequently met with in children, in whom they may be excited through the influence of a dream, but which at other times have no such origin. The condition in question is only induced by the sudden waking of a person.

A very excellent account of sleep drunkenness, in its medico-legal relations, is given by Wharton and Stillé,* who have quoted several interesting cases from German and other authors, which I do not hesitate to transfer to these pages.

"A sentry fell asleep during his watch, and, being suddenly aroused by the officer in command, attacked the latter with his sword, and would have

---

* A Treatise on Medical Jurisprudence, Philadelphia, 1855, p. 120.

(304)

killed him but for the interposition of the by-
standers. The result of the medical examination
was, that the act was involuntary and irresponsible,
being the result of a violent confusion of mind consequent upon the sudden waking from a profound
sleep.

"A day-laborer killed his wife with a wagon-tire,
the blow being struck immediately on his starting
up from a deep sleep from which he was forcibly
awakened. In this case there was collateral evidence that the defendant was seized, on awaking,
with a delusion that a 'woman in white' had
snatched his wife from his side and was carrying
her away, and that his agony of mind was so great
that his whole body was bathed in perspiration.

"A young man, named A. F., about twenty years
of age, was living with his parents in great apparent
harmony, his father and himself being alike distin
guished for their great fondness for hunting. In
consequence of danger from nocturnal attacks, they
were in the habit of taking their arms with them
into their chambers when they went to bed. On
the afternoon of September 1st, 1839, the father and
son having just returned from hunting, their danger
became the subject of particular conversation. The
next day the hunting was repeated, and on their
return, after taking supper with every evidence of
good feeling, they retired for the night, the son to
his own room, and his father and mother to theirs.
Both father and son took their loaded arms with

them. At one o'clock the father got up to go into the entry, and on his return jarred against the door, on which the son instantly sprang up, seized his gun, and discharged it at his father, giving him a fatal wound in the breast, at the same time exclaiming, 'Dog, what do you want here?' The father immediately fell to the ground; and the son, then recognizing him, sank on the floor, crying, 'Oh, Jesus! it is my father!'

"The evidence was that the whole family were subject to great restlessness in their sleep, and that the defendant in particular was affected with a tendency to be easily distressed by dreams, which lasted for about five minutes, on waking, before their effect was entirely dissipated. His own version of the affair was: 'I must have fired the gun in my sleep; it was moonshine, and we were accustomed to talk and walk in our sleep. I recollect hearing something jar; I jumped up, seized my gun, and fired when I heard the noise; I recollect seeing nothing, nor am I conscious of having spoken. The night was so bright that everything could have been seen. I must have been under the delusion that thieves had broken in.' The opinion of the medical experts was, that the act was committed during the condition of sleep drunkenness, and that, accordingly, it was not that of a free and responsible agent.

The same authors quote the following case of Dr. Meister, from Herke's Zeitschrift:

"I was obliged," says the doctor, "to take a jour-

ney of eight miles on a very hot summer's day—my
seat being with my back to the horses, and the sun
directly in my face. On reaching the place of destination, and being very weary and with a slight
headache, I laid myself down, with my clothes on,
on a couch. I fell at once asleep, my head having
slipped under the back of the settee. My sleep was
deep, and, as far as I can recollect, without dreams.
When it became dark, the lady of the house came
with a light into the room. I suddenly awoke, but,
for the first time in my life, without collecting myself. I was seized with a sudden agony of mind,
and, picturing the object which was entering the
house as a specter, I sprang up and seized a stool,
which, in my terror, I would have thrown at the
supposed shade. Fortunately I was recalled to
consciousness by the firmness and tact of the lady
herself, who, with the greatest presence of mind,
succeeded in composing my attention until I was
entirely awakened."

Hoffbauer* relates the particulars of a case which
has passed into the annals of medical jurisprudence
as one of great importance.

"Bernard Schidmaizig awoke suddenly at midnight. At the same moment he saw a frightful
phantom (at least so his imagination depicted it)

---

* Médecine légale relative aux Aliénés et aux Sourds-Muets,
ou les Lois appliquées aux Désordres de l'Intelligence. Traduit de
l'Allemande par A. M. Chambeyron, avec des Notes par MM. Es-
quirol et Itard. Paris, 1827, p. 256.

standing near him.

standing near him. That which appeared to his vision seemed to be a veritable specter; and fear and the darkness of the night prevented him recognizing anything with distinctness. With a feeble voice, he twice called out, 'Who goes there?' He received no answer, and imagined that the apparition was approaching him. Deprived for the instant of his reason, he jumped from his bed, seized a hatchet which he generally kept near him, and with this weapon attacked the imaginary specter. To see this apparition, to cry, 'Who goes there?' to seize the hatchet, were all done in a moment: he had not an instant for reflection. At the first blow the phantom was struck to the earth; Schidmaizig heard a deep groan. This sound, and the noise of the imaginary phantom falling to the ground, fully awakened him; and suddenly the thought struck him that he had assaulted his wife, who slept with him. He threw himself on his knees, raised the head of the wounded person, saw the injury he had inflicted, and the blood which flowed, and with a voice full of anguish cried, 'Susannah! Susannah! come to yourself!' He then called his eldest daughter, aged about eight years—ordered her to see if her mother was recovering, and to tell her grandmother what he had done. It was in reality his wife; and she died the next day from the effects of the blow "

As Hoffbauer remarks, "This man did not enjoy the free use of his senses; he did not know what he saw; he believed that he was repulsing a sudden attack. He very soon recognized the place where he ordinarily slept; it was natural that he should seize his hatchet,—since he had taken the precaution to place it near him,—but the idea of his wife, and of the possibility of having killed her, were the last thoughts that entered his mind."

Seafield* quotes from the Express (London) of January 5th, 1859, the following case of sleep drunkenness:

" Yesterday the Marylebone Police Court was crowded to excess, in consequence of a report which had been circulated, that a woman was in custody for killing her child by throwing it from a first-floor window into the street. The rumor in regard to the murder happily turned out to be untrue; but it will be seen from the subjoined evidence that it was a providential circumstance that the lives of three children were not sacrificed by their mother while acting under the influence of a dream.

"At two o'clock the prisoner, Esther Griggs, was placed at the bar before Mr. Broughton.

" Mr. Lewis, of Ely Place, appeared for her; and Mr. Tubbs, relieving officer of Marylebone, attended on behalf of the board of guardians of the parish, to watch the case.

" The prisoner, who evidently felt the serious situation in which she was placed, was seated during the proceedings.

---

* The Literature and Curiosities of Dreams, etc., London, 1865, vol. ii. p. 332.

"The first witness called was Sergeant Simmons, 20 D, who said, 'At half-past one o'clock this morning, while on duty in East Street, Manchester Square, I heard a female voice exclaim, "Oh, my children! Save my children!" I went to the house, No. 71, from whence the cries proceeded, and the landlord opened the door. I went up-stairs, accompanied by two other constables, and, while making our way to the first floor, I heard the smashing of glass. I knocked at the door, which I found was fastened, and said, "Open it; the police are here." The prisoner, who was in her night-dress, kept on exclaiming, "Save my children!" and at length, after stumbling over something, let me and my brother officers in. When we entered, we found the room in total darkness; and it was only by the aid of our lanterns that we could distinguish anything in the room. On the bed there was a child five years old, and another, three years of age, by her side. Everything in the room was in confusion. She kept crying out, "Where's my baby? Have they caught it? I must have thrown it out of the window." The baby must have been thrown out as I was going up-stairs; for before getting into the room I heard something fall. I left a constable in charge of the prisoner; and I ascertained that the child which had been thrown from the window had been taken to the infirmary of Marylebone Workhouse. She told me she had been dreaming that her little boy had said that the house was on fire, and that what she had done was with the view of preventing her children from being burned to death. I have no doubt,' added the witness, ' that if I and the other constable had not gone to the room all three of the children would have been thrown into the street.'

"Mr. Broughton.—'How long do you suppose the cry of "Oh, save my children!" continued?'

"Witness.—'I should think about five minutes.' (In continuation, he said he went to 38 Harley Street, where the husband lives, in the service of a gentleman, and gave him information of what had occurred. The injured infant was only eighteen months old.)

"By Mr. Lewis.—'From the excited state in which the prisoner was, I did not at the time take her into custody. She went to the infirmary along with her husband, to see how the child was going on, and what hurt it had sustained. I had understood that the surgeon had said it was a species of nightmare which the prisoner was laboring under when the act was committed. The window had not been thrown up. The child was thrust through a pane of glass, the fragments of which fell into the street.'

"Humphreys, 180 D.—'I heard the breaking of glass, and saw what I imagined to be a bundle come out of the window, and, on taking it up, I found it to be a female infant. There was blood running from its temples, and it was insensible. I took it to the infirmary.'

"Pollard, 314 D.—'I heard loud cries of "Oh, save my children!'" and when I was in her room she said, "Has anybody caught my baby Lizzie?" One of the little boys, about three years old, and who was clinging to his mother, had blood upon his clothes. He had upon his breast some marks, which appeared to have been caused by cuts from glass. He left me to take care of the prisoner while he went for her husband. She told me she had no wish to hurt any of her children, and that it was all through a dream.'

"Mr. Henry Tyrwhitt Smith, surgeon of the Marylebone Infirmary, was next called, and said, 'That when the infant was brought to him, soon after one in the morning, he found, upon examining it, that it was suffering from concussion of the brain. It was quite insensible, and decidedly in danger now. The parietal bone is broken, and death might ensue in the event of an effusion of blood on the brain.'

"By Mr. Lewis.—'I cannot say that I have not heard of an instance where parties have committed acts to which a dream had impelled them.'

"Mr. Lewis submitted to the magistrate that there had been no attempt to murder the infant. The prisoner had always evinced a kindly feeling toward her children, and he (the learned gentleman) hoped that the magistrate would allow the husband to have her under his care during the temporary remand which would of course take place The dream under which the act was committed showed that she had not, at the time, any consciousness of what she was doing.

"Mr. Tubbs said he did not attend in the capacity of a prosecutor, but he appeared on behalf of the board of guardians; and he put it to the magistrate whether there would be any objections, under the circumstances, to allow the prisoner to be bailed, her husband being security for her reappearance.

"Mr. Broughton *considered that it would be a most dangerous doctrine to lay down, to say that because a person was dreaming while committing an offense, that they were not culpable for their acts.* A woman, on these grounds, might get up in the middle of the night and cut her husband's throat, and, when brought up for the offense, turn round and say that she had done the act while under the influence of a dream. He (the worthy magistrate) considered the case to be one of a serious nature; and in the event of death ensuing, an inquest would be held on the body. He could not think of taking bail in so serious a case, but would remand the prisoner till Tuesday next, and during her present excited state she would be taken care of in the infirmary.

"The prisoner was then removed to the cells by Ansted, the jailer, sobbing most bitterly.

"The recorder, at the subsequent sessions at the Central Criminal Court, in his address to the grand jury, took a somewhat more rational view of the case than that entertained by Mr. Broughton.

27

"'If the prisoner,' said the recorder, 'really did the act under the idea that it was the best mode of insuring the safety of the child, it appeared to him that, under such circumstances, it would be a question whether the grand jury would be justified in coming to the conclusion that the criminal was guilty of a criminal act.'

"The grand jury threw out the bill."

Several cases of sleep drunkenness have come under my own notice.

A gentleman was roused one night by his wife, who heard the street-door bell ring. He got up, and, without paying attention to what she said, dragged the sheets off of the bed, tore them hurriedly into strips, and proceeded to tie the pieces together. She finally succeeded in bringing him to himself, when he said he thought the house was on fire, and he was providing means for their escape. He did not recollect having had any dream of the kind, but was under the impression that the idea had occurred to him at the instant of his awaking.

Another was suddenly aroused from a sound sleep by the slamming of a window shutter by the wind. He sprang instantly from his bed, and, seizing a chair that was near, hurled it with all his strength against the window. The noise of the breaking of glass fully awakened him. He explained that he imagined some one was trying to get into the house and had let his pistol fall on the floor, thereby producing the noise which had startled him.

A lady informed me that upon one occasion she had gone to bed very tired, but was suddenly startled from her sleep by a voice calling her by name. Without stopping a moment, she arose, put on her shoes and stockings, lit a candle, took a loaded pistol from a shelf near her husband's head, cocked it, and was leaving the room, the pistol in one hand and the candle in the other, when she was seized by her husband. She turned, recognized him at once, and would have fallen to the floor had he not caught her in his arms. Her husband, who slept in the same bed with her, had heard one of the children cry in an adjoining room, and had called her. She, hearing his voice, had partially awakened, but had conceived the idea that he had called to her from another part of the house, where some danger menaced him. She had acted upon this supposition, and was perfectly conscious of every movement she had made.

It does not appear that some persons are more liable to attacks of sleep drunkenness than others. Neither do I know of any means by which its occurrence could be prevented. It is a natural phenomenon, to which all are liable. It is more important in its medico-legal relations than any other.

APPENDIX.

ADDITIONAL OBSERVATIONS RELATIVE TO THE PHYSIOLOGY OF SLEEP.*

SINCE the chapter on the Physiology of Sleep was written, I have, by additional experiments, satisfied myself that the theory then enunciated is correct in every essential particular.

By means of an instrument adapted to show the extent of cerebral pressure, and which I first described nearly two years ago, I have been enabled to arrive at very positive results. In every instance the pressure was lessened during sleep and was increased during wakefulness. The experiments were performed upon dogs and rabbits. Briefly, the instrument consists of a brass tube, which is screwed into a round hole made in the skull with a trephine. Both ends of this tube are open, but into the upper is screwed another brass tube, the lower end of which is closed by a piece of very thin sheet india-rubber, and the upper end with a brass cap, into

---

* See New York Medical Gazette and Quarterly Journal of Psychological Medicine and Medical Jurisprudence, January, 1869, p. 47.

(317)

which is fastened a glass tube. This inner arrangement contains colored water, and to the glass tube a scale is affixed.

This second brass tube is screwed into the first, till the thin rubber presses upon the dura mater and the level of the colored water stands at 0, which is in the middle of the scale. Now, when the animal goes to sleep, the liquid falls in the tube, showing that the cerebral pressure has been diminished, —an event which can only take place in consequence of a reduction in the quantity of blood circulating through the brain. As soon as the animal awakes, the liquid rises at once. Nothing can exceed the conclusiveness of experiments of this character. No mere theorizing can avail against them.

Published by J. B. LIPPINCOTT & CO., Philadelphia.

Will be sent by Mail, post-paid, on receipt of price.

A TREATISE ON THE PRACTICE OF MEDICINE.

By GEORGE B. WOOD, M.D., LL.D., President of the College of
Physicians of Philadelphia; Emeritus Professor of the Theory
and Practice of Medicine in the University of Pennsylvania;
one of the authors of the Dispensatory of the United States of
America, etc. Sixth Edition. In two volumes 8vo. Sheep.
Price $11.00.

Eight years have passed since the appearance of the fifth edition
of this well-known and highly valued work, a period within which
many and great advances have been made in medicine, so that the
year spent by the author exclusively in bringing this treatise up to
the present state of science was none too long for such a task.
Some of the introductory chapters on general pathology have been
modified, in accordance with the views of modern observers, descriptions of a large number of new affections have been introduced in
their proper connection, and much new matter relating to special
diseases has been inserted in the form of foot-notes. Altogether,
two hundred pages have been added to the present edition. The
work is too well known and too highly prized throughout the country to need any praise from us.—*Boston Med. and Surg. Journal.*

ELEMENTS OF HUMAN ANATOMY: General, Descriptive, and Practical.

By T. G. RICHARDSON, M.D., Professor of Anatomy in the Medi-
cal Department of the University of Louisiana. SECOND EDI-
TION. Carefully Revised, and Illustrated by nearly Three
Hundred Engravings. One vol. 8vo. Cloth. Price $6.00.

This is a full-sized octavo volume of 671 pages; published in excellent style. Its illustrations are well executed, and, as a whole,
it constitutes one of the best text-books on anatomy that we have
seen.—*Chicago Med. Examiner.*

ANGULAR CURVATURE OF THE SPINE.

Contributions to the Pathology, Diagnosis, and Treatment of
Angular Curvature of the Spine. By BENJAMIN LEE, M.D.
Illustrated. Tinted paper. 12mo. Extra Cloth. Price $1.25.

This is the title of a very excellent book containing several essays
on the above subject. The grand object of the work is to draw the
attention of the profession to the development of mechanical Therapeutics, particularly with reference to Pott's Disease. * * * We
hope the profession will resort to this publication for information,
since it contains valuable knowledge, founded on very careful observations.—*St. Louis Med. Reporter.*

ANSTIE ON EPIDEMICS.

Notes on Epidemics; for the Use of the Public. By FRANCIS ED-
MUND ANSTIE, M.D., F.R.C.P., Senior Assistant Physician to
the Westminster Hospital. 12mo. Cloth. Price $1.00.

This is an expansion of an article by Dr. Austie which originally
appeared in the *British Quarterly Review*. It was designed to furnish "information which may assist the non-medical public to do
their part in the work of preventing" those epidemic diseases which
are the scourge of our cities. The little volume deserves a wide
circulation.—*Chicago Medical Journal.*

THE COMMON NATURE OF EPIDEMICS, and their Rela-
tions to Climate and Civilization.

Also, Remarks on Contagion and Quarantine. From Writings and
Official Reports. By SOUTHWOOD SMITH, M.D., Physician to
the London Fever Hospital, etc. etc. Edited by T. BAKER, Esq.
12mo. Cloth. Price $1.50.

A TREATISE ON THERAPEUTICS AND PHARMACOL-
OGY OR MATERIA MEDICA.

By GEORGE B. WOOD, M.D. Third Edition. Revised and Enlarged.
Two vols. 8vo.

INTESTINAL OBSTRUCTION.

By WM. BRINTON, M.D., F.R.S. Edited by THOMAS BUZZARD,
M.D., Lond. Illustrated. One vol. 12mo. Price $1.50.

EMOTIONAL DISORDERS.

A Treatise on Emotional Disorders of the Sympathetic System of
Nerves. By WILLIAM MURRAY, M.D., M.R.C.P., etc. London,
12mo. Cloth. Price $1.50.

SHOCK.

A Practical Treatise on Shock after Surgical Operations and Injuries, with especial reference to Shock after Railway Accidents.
By EDWIN MORRIS, M.D., etc. One vol. 12mo. Cloth.

PRACTICAL ANATOMY.

A new arrangement of the London Dissector, with numerous Modifications and Additions. By D. HAYES AGNEW, M.D., etc.
SECOND EDITION. REVISED. 12mo. Cloth.

SLEEP AND ITS DERANGEMENTS.

By WILLIAM A. HAMMOND, M.D. One vol. 12mo. [*In Press.*]

Life: its Nature, Varieties, and Phenomena.

By LEO H. GRINDON, Lecturer on Botany at the Royal School of Medicine, Manchester; author of "Emblems," "Figurative Language," etc. First American edition. 1 vol. 8vo. $2.25

The object of this work is twofold. First, it is proposed to give a popular account of the phenomena which indicate the presence of that mysterious sustaining force we denominate Life, or Vitality, and of the laws which appear to govern their manifestation; secondly, will be considered those Spiritual or Emotional and Intellectual States, which collectively constitute the essential history of our temporal lives, rendering existence either pleasurable or painful. The inquiry will thus embrace all the most interesting and instructive subjects alike of physiology and psychology: the constitution and functions of the bodies in which we dwell; the delights which attend the exercise of the intellect and affections; the glory and loveliness of the works of God, will all come under notice, and receive their fitting meed of illustration. Especially will the practical value and interest of life be pointed out: the unity and fine symmetry of the True, the Beautiful, and the Good, the poetry of "common things," and the intimate dependence of the whole upon Him in whom "we live, and move, and have our being." * * * * *

To those who care for the illustration which physical science casts upon the science of mind, and upon the truths of Revelation, there will probably be much that is both novel and inviting. In fact, it has been sedulously aimed to show how intimate and striking is the relation of human knowledges, and how grand is the harmony of things natural and divine. * * * There has been no hesitation in dealing with some of the most sacred of topics. The physical and the spiritual worlds are in such close connection, that to attempt to treat philosophically of either of them apart from the other, is to divorce what God has joined together. * * * Science without religion is empty and unvital. True wisdom, finding the whole world expressive of God, calls upon us to walk at all times and in all places, in the worship and reverent contemplation of Him.—*Preface.*

Mosaics of Life.

Illustrative of the various Epochs of Human Life—Betrothal, Wedded Life, Babyhood, Youth, Single Life, Old Age. By MRS. ELIZABETH A. THURSTON. 12mo. $2.00.

A short acquaintance with it will secure it a place among those choice volumes which are to be found in every library, and which are esteemed of more value than their weight in gold. It is splendidly printed on delicately tinted paper, and is in all respects a charming volume.—*Boston Journal.*

As a volume for the parlor-table, as a book of reference to the vast realms of thought and emotion, it will be found full of information, suggestion, and inspiration.—*Boston Transcript.*

Hymns of Praise.

Compiled by HENRY A. BOARDMAN, D.D. Fourth Edition. 16mo. Roan. Price, $1.25.

VALUABLE AND INSTRUCTIVE WORKS

RECENTLY PUBLISHED BY

J. B. LIPPINCOTT & CO., Philadelphia.

FIVE YEARS WITHIN THE GOLDEN GATE.

By ISABELLE SAXON. Crown 8vo. Fine stamped cloth. $2.50
"This volume is instructive and entertaining."—*The Press.*

A SUMMER IN ICELAND.

By C. W. PAIJKULL. Translated by M. R. BARNARD, B.A. With map and numerous illustrations. 8vo. Cloth. $5.00.

AMONG THE ARABS.

A Narrative of Adventures in Algeria. By G. NAPHEGYI, M.D., etc., author of "The Album of Language," "History of Hungary," "La Cueva Del Diablo," etc. With Portrait of Author. 12mo. Tinted paper. Fine cloth, beveled boards. $1.75.

"The author describes a journey in Algeria, in which he had peculiar facilities for observing and studying the habits, customs, and peculiarities of the people of that land—of whom but comparatively little is known. He has made one of the most interesting books of travel which have been issued for a long time."—*Boston Journal.*

MORTE DARTHUR.

SIR THOMAS MALORY's Book of King Arthur and his Noble Knights of the Round Table. The original Edition of Caxton revised for modern use, with an Introduction by SIR EDWARD STRACHEY, Bart. THE GLOBE EDITION. Square 12mo. Tinted paper. Cloth. $1.75.

CURIOUS MYTHS.

Curious Myths of the Middle Ages. By S. BARING GOULD. Second Series. 12mo. Illustrated. Tinted paper. Fine cloth. $2.50.

LIVES OF THE ENGLISH CARDINALS,

Including Historical Notices of the Papal Court, from Nicholas Breakspear (Pope Adrian IV.) to Thomas Wolsey, Cardinal Legate. By FOLKESTONE WILLIAMS, author of "The Court and Times of James I.," etc. Two vols. 8vo. Cloth. $12.00.

AB-SA-RA-KA, HOME OF THE CROWS.

Being the Experience of an Officer's Wife on the Plains: marking the vicissitudes of peril and pleasure during the first occupation of the Powder River route to Montana, 1866–67, and the Indian hostility thereto: with outlines of the natural features and resources of the land; tables of distances, and other aids to the traveler. Gathered from observation and other reliable sources. 12mo. Illustrated with maps and wood engravings. Tinted paper. Fine cloth. $2.00.

NEW AMERICA.

By WILLIAM HEPWORTH DIXON, Editor of "The Athenæum," and author of "The Holy Land," "William Penn," etc. With Illustrations from Original Photographs. Third Edition. Complete in one volume, Crown Octavo. Printed on tinted paper. Extra Cloth. Price $2.75.

In these graphic volumes Mr. Dixon sketches American men and women, sharply, vigorously, and truthfully, under every aspect. The smart Yankee, the grave politician, the senate and the stage, the pulpit and the prairie, loafers and philanthropists, crowded streets and the howling wilderness, the saloon and the boudoir, with women everywhere at full length—all passes on before us in some of the most vivid and brilliant pages ever written.—*Dublin University Magazine.*

ELEMENTS OF ART CRITICISM.

A Text-book for Schools and Colleges, and a Hand-book for Amateurs and Artists. By G. W. SAMSON, D.D., President of Columbian College, Washington, D. C. Second Edition. Crown 8vo. Cloth. Price $3.50. Abridged Edition $1.75.

This work comprises a Treatise on the Principles of Man's Nature as addressed by Art, together with a Historic survey of the Methods of Art Execution in the departments of Drawing, Sculpture, Architecture, Painting, Landscape Gardening, and the Decorative Arts. The *Round Table* says: "The work is incontestably one of great as well as unique value."

THE HISTORY OF ART.

By PROFESSOR WILHELM LUBKE. Translated by F. E. BUNNETT, translator of Grimm's "Life of Michael Angelo," etc. With 415 illustrations. Two vols. imperial 8vo. Beautifully printed from Old Faced type on toned paper, and handsomely bound in cloth.

TERRA MARIÆ; or, Threads of Maryland Colonial History.

By EDWARD D. NEILL, one of the Secretaries of the President of the United States. 12mo. Extra Cloth. Price $2.00.

COMING WONDERS, expected between 1867 and 1875.

By the Rev. M. BAXTER, author of "The Coming Battle." One vol. 12mo. Cloth. Price $1.00.

CPSIA information can be obtained
at www.ICGtesting.com
Printed in the USA
LVHW05s2313171018
593997LV00019B/1048/P